T0320868

Essential Skills for Physiotherapists

Essential Skills for Physiotherapists

A Personal and Professional Development Framework

Edited by

David Clancy, MSc, BSc, HC, MISCP, CORU

Sports Medicine Specialist and Consultant

Co-Founder and Director
The Nxt Level Group
Dublin, Ireland

Co-Founder and Director
Hauora
Dublin, Ireland

Co-Founder and Director
The Learning Physiotherapist
Dublin, Ireland

Stuart Porter, PhD, BSc, GradDip, PgCAP, CertMHS, SFHEA, MLACP, MCSP, HCPC

Lecturer in Physiotherapy
University of Salford
Manchester, UK

Health and Care Professions Council Registered
Senior Fellow Higher Education Academy
Expert Witness
Manchester, UK

Jeff Konin, PhD, ATC, PT, FACSM, FNATA, FNAP

Clinical Professor and Director of DAT Program
Florida International University
Miami, Florida, USA

Amelia J. H. Arundale, PhD, DPT, BSc, PT

Senior Performance Therapist and Biomechanist
Washington Wizards
Washington DC, USA

Adjunct Professor
Ichan School of Medicine
Mount Sinai Health System
New York, USA

Grant Downie, OBE, GradDip, GradDip, MCSP, HCPC

Medical and Performance Solutions Consultant
Elite Human Performance
Isle of Arran, Scotland, UK

Varying sporting organisations/brands and national
governing bodies globally
Isle of Arran, Scotland, UK

Ciaran Dunne, MSc, MSc, BSc, PGCert, MISCP, CORU

Health & Performance Specialist and Consultant

Clinical Specialist Physiotherapist
Mater Private Network
Dublin, Ireland

Co-Founder and Director
Hauora
Dublin, Ireland

Co-Founder and Director
The Learning Physiotherapist
Dublin, Ireland

ELSEVIER

© 2025, Elsevier Limited. All rights are reserved, including those for text and data mining, AI training, and similar technologies.

Publisher's note: *Elsevier* takes a neutral position with respect to territorial disputes or jurisdictional claims in its published content, including in maps and institutional affiliations.

No part of this publication may be reproduced or transmitted in any form or by any means, electronic or mechanical, including photocopying, recording, or any information storage and retrieval system, without permission in writing from the publisher. Details on how to seek permission, further information about the Publisher's permissions policies and our arrangements with organizations such as the Copyright Clearance Center and the Copyright Licensing Agency, can be found at our website: www.elsevier.com/permissions.

This book and the individual contributions contained in it are protected under copyright by the Publisher (other than as may be noted herein).

Notices

Practitioners and researchers must always rely on their own experience and knowledge in evaluating and using any information, methods, compounds or experiments described herein. Because of rapid advances in the medical sciences, in particular, independent verification of diagnoses and drug dosages should be made. To the fullest extent of the law, no responsibility is assumed by Elsevier, authors, editors or contributors for any injury and/or damage to persons or property as a matter of products liability, negligence or otherwise, or from any use or operation of any methods, products, instructions, or ideas contained in the material herein.

ISBN: 978-0-443-11128-0

Content Strategist: Andrae Akeh
Content Project Manager: Tapajyoti Chaudhuri
Cover Design: Hitchen Miles
Marketing Manager: Deborah J. Watkins

Printed in India.
Last digit is the print number: 9 8 7 6 5 4 3 2 1

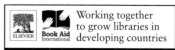

CONTENTS

First, I'd like to thank David, in particular, and the editors for inviting me to write this foreword, for what I see as a hugely important book for many in the industry, be them young or old, experienced or new in their career.

This is not a self-help book per se; however, by reading, reflecting and then implementing the lessons held in the following pages you are making an investment in your own personal development. In turn, this will improve the quality and impact of your work output and the sense of belonging and enjoyment in what you do.

Over my working career I have really learnt and observed the old adage that it is not the quality of the idea that is important. The true impact of the idea comes from the quality of the delivery or implementation. We shouldn't be seeking to claim credit for ideas; we should be feeling energy and contentment from an idea well delivered.

To deliver well we need to be intentional and well prepared. We are not taught in the traditional curriculums to listen, to speak up or to have courageous conversations. So my hope is that you will learn things and gain insights that you can benefit from across life, not simply in your professional work settings. This book brings together real-life experiences and academic thought, from a wide cross-section of the industry. Leaders in their own fields, often most lauded for their technical knowledge. And whilst these technical and clinical skills matter, when everyone has those it's the personal touch that makes all the difference.

Never has there been a more relevant time for this book. After the Covid-19 pandemic there is ever more focus on health in society and individuals searching for more meaning in life, looking for community around us and seeking more authentic connectedness. In this context, what we should always understand is that we are human beings interacting with other human beings. Human beings that are connected to one another. And at the heart of that is emotional intelligence and the way that we communicate with each other. Ultimately, we are here to serve, and to do this best we need to be the best versions of ourselves, especially outside of the technical dimension of our work.

Perhaps for a moment it is worth reflecting on where I come from and where my perspective on this book could be relevant.

Mine is a different story.

Neither a practitioner nor an academic.

No fledgling sporting career.

No serious injury in my youth that led me to meet physiotherapy.

But bound to this industry to do good and serve people.

And provide opportunities for all stakeholders in what we do.

Those who know me will often hear me speak historically about talent. I have spent nearly 20 years in the identification of, the recruitment of, the development of and then the team blending of talent. Within this search for and celebration of talent, my thinking evolved initially to recognise the importance and impact of cognitive diversity. Diversity not just of background, geography or education but also the celebration of different thinking. Not necessarily looking to find voices from outside the box, but as Matthew Syed talks about in *Rebel Ideas*, looking to the corners of the box and challenging the concept of groupthink or leader-idea confluences. The key is to bring more intelligence and experience to the room for the benefit of the patient or athlete.

In the past 24 to 36 months my thinking has been challenged even more. Thinking beyond talent on an individual basis and thinking more of the power of community and the challenge of creating interdisciplinarity in a sports medicine and sports performance context. Emotional intelligence at a singular level and then collective team level is now what I see as the difference maker, the potentiality for satisfying and high-performing teams to live and breathe. To foster this, all of us must challenge ourselves to think about having a small sense of self. Self-awareness is a fundamental assumption in allowing this to happen.

In the past month I have spent time observing and investigating communication models in high-performance sport, from Michelin star kitchens to special operations teams in the military to conductor-less orchestras. What I have sought to try and understand, in all these settings, are the following challenges.

- **Trust:** How does the leader (with or without authority) inspire trust? Why is its existence so important? How does mutual trust generate confidence and creative freedom?
- **Communication:** What is the true difference between feedback and criticism, and how does it show up? How do you get the best out of a high-functioning team? How can effective communication create a positive climate in the organisation?
- **Empowerment/shared ownership:** How does the leader build environments where all of us can be equally motivated and feel an equal stake in the shared goal of a great performance? Understanding of role – ensuring clarity and that there is no such thing as a minor role – there can be no passengers.
- **Vision:** How can the leader inspire and impart a vision without stifling the creativity of their colleagues? Effective leadership = direction, not control. How a leader can learn from their colleagues, and how this can develop their vision.
- **Risk:** How does risk increase reward, bring the team together and inspire greater achievement? How can the leader engender a culture of freedom and risk-taking?

My early conclusions are that courage is at the heart of this. You need to step forward, be brave, embrace the here and now and continually invest in yourself. Being self-aware is the next step, actively building and developing skills such as the ones detailed in this book. We can then build through collaboration with others (equipped with similar skills) the continuum of enhanced flow and excitement in our work:

Cohesion > synchronicity > collective effervescence

I feel a deep responsibility to advocate for the sports medicine and performance sciences community, and to help create an environment for those entering the industry to flourish in. After reading the pages ahead, I encourage you to challenge yourself to listen more and ask better questions. Keep being curious, engaged and present. Try to make informed decisions, be aware of your emotions and proactively find ways to develop trusted and meaningful relationships. This is life and this is being.

Michael Davison MBA, MA, BA
Football Research Group; Performance Support and Athlete
Care for Brooklyn Nets, Houston Texans and Chelsea FC,
London, UK

It is so useful to be able to read about physiotherapists' personal experiences and the professional frameworks that they are working in to enhance your knowledge and help you in future decision-making.

Gary Lewin BSc (Hons) Dip Phys, MCSP
Director at Lewin Sports Injury Clinic; Current Head of Performance Services
at Arsenal Women's Football Club; former Arsenal FC Head Physiotherapist,
Director of Physiotherapy Services English FA and England National Football
Team, and former Head of Medical and Sports Science Services West Ham.

I am thrilled about this book. Along with being a master clinician, one must also excel in the most crucial aspect of patient care: the soft skills. This is for everyone who wants to get better at these.

Johnny Owens BS, MPT
CEO and Director of Clinical Research & Education for Owens Recovery
Science; former Chief of Human Performance Optimization at the Center for the
Intrepid at San Antonio Military Medical Center; Consultant to many NFL, NBA
and NCAA organisations

I am a firm believer that the most important skills a clinician can have are their ability to listen and perform a sound clinical evaluation, alongside a culture of lifelong learning and reflection. Ideally, we learn from other's mistakes and experiences; however, we have to confront our own mistakes and at times go through painful learning, rather than denial. I am sure this book will provide very valuable lessons.

Dr Phil Batty MB ChB, MRCGP, PG, Dip (SEM), FFSEM
Consultant in Sport and Exercise Medicine with Cleveland Clinic; Chief
Medical Officer for Middlesex Cricket, Consultant in Sport and Exercise Medicine
for English National Ballet, President of Independent Doctors Federation;
former Deputy Club Doctor at Manchester United, Head of Sports Medicine at
Manchester City, former Senior Team Doctor for the England Rugby Team, and
former Consultant in Sports and Exercise Medicine for Isokinetic Medical Group

I am delighted to provide a testimonial for this book which highlights the importance of soft skills as well as hard clinical expertise. This guide provides vital information for physiotherapists aiming to enhance their soft skills, including communication, leadership and wellness. It is well recognised that combining clinical expertise with these soft skills leads to improved patient outcomes and I would regard this guide as essential reading for all clinicians aiming to improve their care.

Professor John M. O'Byrne
Abraham Colles Chair in Trauma and Orthopaedic Surgery, Royal College
of Surgeons in Ireland; Clinical Director & Consultant Orthopaedic Surgeon,
National Orthopaedic Hospital Cappagh; Honorary Orthopaedic Surgeon, Ireland
Senior Soccer Team – Football Association of Ireland; former UEFA Chief Medical
Officer EURO 2020 Dublin

David Clancy   ▪   Ciaran Dunne   ▪   Ashley James

'The important thing is not to stop questioning. Curiosity has its own reason for existing. One cannot help but be in awe when he contemplates the mysteries of eternity, of life, of the marvellous structure of reality. It is enough if one tries merely to comprehend a little of this mystery every day. Never lose a holy curiosity.'
– Albert Einstein, physicist and founder of the Theory of Relativity

It was never just about the technical and clinical skill set.

What separates the best in healthcare is the other stuff. Human skills. Interpersonal skills. Life skills. People skills. Soft skills. Real skills, as Seth Godin calls them.

These skills are harder to learn and even harder to master, but also they are not taught to us as undergraduates or postgraduates with the same intensity or depth as traditional physiotherapy. These skills, such as the ability to communicate effectively, leverage curiosity and creativity, network with intention, navigate adversity, negotiate with influence, build trust with empathy, manage and lead one and another and work in a team, are essential in the development of self, clinical outcomes and more broadly the overall success and influence of the profession.

For us, soft skills are the difference maker. That's why The Learning Physiotherapist was created a few years ago, an online learning and mentoring community with world-renowned mentors that focuses purely on the soft skills.

There is no doubt that building a rapport and connection with a patient from the first moment not only creates meaning for the individual in front of you but also, as evidence demonstrates, clearly leads to better patient outcomes. The technical and clinical skills matter, of course, but without the platform of connection with the patient, they become null and void. Listening, asking better questions, being engaged and present, making shared decisions and being emotionally intelligent – this is what can really help. When we think about people we admire (in any walk of life), it is how they interact and communicate that speaks volumes. As the old saying goes, you remember less what people did and much more how they made you feel.

The practitioners, mentors and leaders who these contributing authors have worked with are world-class, and they clearly marry the clinical with the soft skills. It is always a patient-first approach, starting from a place of empathy (like a design-thinking methodology).

This book aims to unpack the essential skills for physiotherapists, to take you as the reader on a journey through wellbeing, articulating purpose and values, network building, habit building, goals, motivation, high-performance, interdisciplinarity, building a personal brand, life-work alignment and mental fitness, amongst many other topics. This is a highly tactical, practical book with opportunities for reflective practice and key takeaways you can act on immediately. There are unique stories from multiple high-performers sharing their triumphs, setbacks and lessons for how to improve and develop.

Feel free to pick this book up and skip between chapters or from cover to cover in order. Both methods will work. The key thing is to enjoy it. The combined experience in this book is truly world-class, with contributing authors from around the world representing a diverse range of cultural backgrounds. They have made mistakes and learnt from them and are sharing those lessons with you. We ideated this book with the intention for it to be wide-ranging and eclectic, with inputs from sports medicine, private practice, public and hospital care, academia, governing bodies and high-performance sport. We intended to bring together the needle-movers and thought leaders who recognise the power of being aware, present and open to continual learning and development, coupled with the practicality of applying these skills at work and home. And we believe we have been successful with this intention.

Enjoy this.

David Clancy, MSc, BSc, HC, MISCP, CORU
Sports Medicine Specialist and Consultant
Co-Founder and Director
The Nxt Level Group, Dublin, Ireland;
Co-Founder and Director
Hauora, Dublin, Ireland;
Co-Founder and Director
The Learning Physiotherapist, Dublin, Ireland

Stuart Porter, PhD, BSc, GradDip, PgCAP, CertMHS, SFHEA, MLACP, MCSP, HCPC
Lecturer in Physiotherapy
University of Salford
Health and Care Professions Council
    Registered
Senior Fellow Higher Education Academy
Expert Witness, Manchester, UK

Jeff Konin, PhD, ATC, PT, FACSM, FNATA, FNAP
Clinical Professor & Director of DAT Program
Florida International University
Miami, Florida, USA

Amelia J. H. Arundale, PhD, DPT, BSc, PT
Senior Performance Therapist and Biomecha-
    nist at the Washington Wizards
Washington DC, USA;
Adjunct Professor at the Ichan School of
    Medicine at Mount Sinai Health System
New York, NY, USA

Grant Downie, OBE, GradDip, GradDip, MCSP, HCPC
Medical and Performance Solutions Consultant
Elite Human Performance, Varying sporting
    organisations/brands and national govern-
    ing bodies globally
Isle of Arran, Scotland, UK

Ciaran Dunne, MSc, MSc, BSc, PGCert, MISCP, CORU
Health & Performance Specialist and Consultant
Clinical Specialist Physiotherapist
Mater Private Network, Dublin, Ireland;
Co-Founder and Director
Hauora, Dublin, Ireland;
Co-Founder and Director
The Learning Physiotherapist, Dublin, Ireland

Deepak Agnihotri, MSc, MSc, BSc MHCPC MCSP
Director of Allied Health Professionals
Greater Manchester Mental Health NHS
    Foundation Trust
Greater Manchester, UK

Steph Allen, DPT, PT, OCS
Physical Therapist and Performance Coach
Founder of ACLResolve
LLC
Co-Founder of Clinical Athlete
New York, USA

Ritchie Barber, PLY, BSc
Physiotherapist in Sport
Lecturer in Physiotherapy
University of Salford
Para Football Physiotherapist at the Football
    Association
Worsley Physiotherapy and Sports Injury
    Clinic
Salford, UK

Evangelos Benatos, BSc
Head Physiotherapist of Olympiacos
    Basketball Club
Physiotherapist of the Greek Basketball
    National Team
Athens, Greece

Matthew Bruno, B ExSci, DPT
Physiotherapist and Clinical Placement
    Co-Ordinator at Eltham Physiotherapy &
    Sports Injuries
APA Mentor for the Australian Physiotherapy
    Association
Melbourne, Australia

David Cosgrave, MSD, MSc, BSc
Senior Director Sports Medicine and High
    Performance
Orlando City SC
Major League Soccer
Florida, USA

Michael Davison, MBA, MA, BA
Football Research Group
Performance Support and Athlete Care for
  Brooklyn Nets,
Houston Texans and Chelsea F.C.,
London, UK

Chris Desmond, BPhty, PGCert, MMgmt
Lead Physiotherapist/Health & Injury
  Prevention Consultant
North City Physiotherapy/Self-employed
  Consultant
Wellington, New Zealand

Wayne Diesel, PhD, BSc, BSc
Scientific Advisory Board Member
Euleria Health
Holywell, Wales, UK

Darren Finnegan, BSc, NMP, MSCP
Sports Specialist Physio/First Contact
  Practitioner
Director
Pro Health Physio NE
Chair
North East Musculoskeletal Society
FCP
Connect Health - South Tyneside MSK.
Associate Lecturer
Northumbria University
Newcastle Upon Tyne, UK

Colm Fuller, MPhty, BSc, BSc, MISCP, CORU
Head of Physiotherapy
UPMC Sports Surgery Clinic
Dublin, Ireland

Ludovica Gagliardi, MSc, BSc
MSK Sport Physiotherapist
Bologna, Italy

Andreas Gatzoulis, BSc
Physiotherapist
Head of Performance
Olympiacos BC
Piraeus, Greece

Phil Glasgow, PhD, MTh, MRes, PGDip, BSc, FFSEM, PT
Head of Performance Support
High Performance Unit
Irish Rugby Football Union
Dublin, Ireland

Carl Gombrich, Professor
Dean
The London Interdisciplinary School
London, UK

Ian Horsley, Professor, PhD, MCSP, MMACP CSCS
Athlete Health Lead Physiotherapist UK
  Sports Institute
Clinical Director Back In Action
  Rehabilitation Ltd
Wakefield, UK;
Hon Professor
University of Salford
School of Health and Society
Manchester, UK

Ashley James, MS, BSc
Director of Practice and Development
Chartered Society of Physiotherapy
Holywell, Wales, UK

Chris Jones, Dr/Consultant in SEM/MBBS, MRCGP, FFSEM
Consultant in Sport & Exercise Medicine
Sports Medicine & Orthopaedic
  Rehabilitation
Isokinetic Medical Group
London, UK

Derek Lawrance, DAT, ATC
Athletic Trainer
United States Soccer Federation
Men's National Team
Mission Viejo
California, USA

Chrystal Lynch, BSc, PT, RPT
Physiotherapist
Christ Church, Barbados

Ana Mali, MSc, BSc, HCPC, PhD (pursuing)
Assistant
Institute for Kinesiology Research
Science and Research Centre Koper
  (ZRS Koper)
Koper, Slovenia
Vrije Universiteit Brussels (VUB)
Brussels, Belgium

Marita Marshall, MSc, BSc, PT
Physiotherapist & Clinic Owner
Physiotherapy & Optimal Performance
    Services (POPS)
Bridgetown, Barbados

Sergio Martin-Acuna, MS, LAT, ATC
Lead Performance and Rehab Specialist
Orlando City SC
Florida, USA

Jacopo Mattaini, PT, DPT, SCS
Hospital for Special Surgery
Sports Medicine Institute
New York, USA

Roisin McNulty, M.Phty, BSc
Physiotherapist (Titled SP & MSK)
BioInnovate Ireland Fellow 2023-2024
Galway, Ireland

Steve Miller, MSc MACP, BSc
Senior GB Physiotherapist
UK Sports Institute
Chairman of North East Musculoskeletal
    Society (NEMS)
Founder & Mentor in Grow Physio Academy
Birmingham, UK

Chris Morgan, MSc, BSc
Lead Performance Physiotherapist at Liver-
    pool Football Club & Founder/Director of
    Rehab 4 Performance Sports Injury Clinic
Liverpool, UK

Mary O'Keefe, PhD, MSc, BSc
School of Public Health
Physiotherapy and Sports Sciences
University College Dublin
Belfield, Dublin;
European Pain Federation EFIC
Brussels, Belgium

Emmanuel Ovola, MSc, BSc
MSK Physiotherapist
Cultural Health Club
London, UK

Federico Picchetti, MSc, BSc, PGDip
Sport Physiotherapist
Bologna FC
Medical Team
Bologna, Italy

Paolo Policastri, MSc SEM, PT, D.O., MSc Ost
Head Physiotherapist
Medical Department
Parma Calcio Women (1st Team)
Parma, Italy

Barbara Sanders, PT, PhD, SCS, FAPTA
Professor and Chair
Department of Physical Therapy
Associate Dean
College of Health Professions
Texas State University
San Marcos, Texas, USA

Filippo Siragusa, PT, OMT
Physiotherapist
Sports Physiotherapy
YouCare Med
Monza, Italy

Paul Stevens, BSc
First Contact and MSK Physiotherapist
Pure Physiotherapy Associated
The Learning Physiotherapist
Cheshire, UK

Kasper Thornton, BSc, GradDip
Physiotherapist
Director of Human Performance FC
Nordsjælland
Right to Dream Group
Denmark

Nicol van Dyk, Dr/BSc, MSc, PhD
Assistant Professor (Ad Astra Fellow)
School of Public Health
Physiotherapy and Sport Science
University College Dublin
Dublin, Ireland

Evert Verhagen, Dr., Professor
Department Public and Occupational Health
Amsterdam UMC
Amsterdam, Netherlands

Nick Worth, MSc, BSc, MCSP, FSOMM
Consultant Sports Performance Physiotherapist
Chair of the Society of Musculoskeletal
    Medicine (SOMM)
Lecturer - University of Salford Non-Medical
    prescribing Programme
Manchester, UK

Wellbeing

CHAPTER 1

Your Wellbeing

Ludovica Gagliardi ▪ Nick Worth

> *'The mind and body are intimately connected. Taking care of one is essential for taking care of the other.'*
>
> Dr Andrew Huberman, neuroscientist and host of the 'Huberman Lab podcast', 2022

CHAPTER OUTLINE

Introduction	Burnout
A Definition for Wellbeing	Five Key Takeaways
Individual Wellbeing	Five Self-Directed Reflections
Influencing Your Wellbeing	

Introduction

As is widely acknowledged, two key inherent strengths of physiotherapists are empathy and enthusiasm. With empathy we, as physiotherapists, can build trust and craft relationships, and through enthusiasm we can inspire our patients. We offer hope and aspirations for improvement – either through rehabilitation or by simply listening and supporting people by allowing them to share their experiences.

Seeing progress and development in patients serves as the lifeblood that keeps physiotherapists motivated and inspired. But in order to help others, we give a little piece of ourselves away. To be able to assist others, we need to ensure that we take sufficient care of ourselves first.

Just think of the safety information demonstration that is given on every flight before take-off – 'Fit your own oxygen mask first before helping others'. In lifesaving/lifeguard training, the mantra has always been to ensure your own safety before attempting to save another person. There would be no logic in there being two casualties as opposed to one, would there? This message is profound and should resonate with us. In order to be most effective in supporting others, we must support ourselves and specifically maximise our wellbeing wherever possible.

If you have ever gotten a snippet or a sense of burnout towards the end of a busy day, and if this repeats itself each week for a sustained period, our ability to maintain empathy and enthusiasm can substantially wane. We will come back to recognition of therapist burnout later in the chapter, but we first need to establish what wellbeing means for each of us.

A Definition for Wellbeing

Health has been defined as 'a state of complete physical, mental and social wellbeing and not the mere absence of disease or infirmity'. According to the World Health Organization (WHO), wellbeing is key to being healthy. So, what exactly is it?

Many researchers have attempted to provide a complete definition of wellbeing and categorise its various aspects. Let's look at some of them.

Wellbeing is seen as an umbrella term under which there are many factors playing a role. Lawton (1983) reported that behavioural competence, perceived quality of life, psychological wellbeing and objective/external environments are key aspects. Additionally, La Placa *et al.* (2013), agreeing with previous work from Knight & McNaught (2011), have set broader categories of wellbeing, such as individual wellbeing, family wellbeing, community wellbeing and societal wellbeing, which all have subcategories that influence each other.

Appreciating that wellbeing is quite a broad and complex concept is critical. By doing so we are able to recognise and reflect on the many factors that play a role and could affect our health.

Firstly, let's look at individual wellbeing … because being able to improve this will positively affect your professional career, among many other aspects of your life.

Individual Wellbeing

Individual wellbeing is multidimensional, and holistic, commonly known as whole person even. It includes physical, mental, social and occupational pillars. These can each be influenced by one another, and subjective or objective circumstances, such as your own experience of financial wellbeing and career, or your social environment.

When considering your own individual wellbeing, the first thing to reflect on is understanding what you have, what you need and how you want to achieve it. A useful concept and tool to find out these key aspects is the Japanese Ikigai model.

Ikigai seems to be the reason why in Japan, and especially on a small island called Okinawa, there are more people over the age of 100 years old (per 100,000 citizens) than anywhere else in the world; this is where people not only live longer but also have fewer diseases such as cancer or cardiovascular issues, age better, have a higher activity level until later in life and have reduced risk of senile dementia compared to the rest of the world (Gavrilova & Gavrilov, 2012; Willcox *et al.*, 2007, 2014).

Ikigai has been translated as 'a reason for being', 'the aim of your life' and 'the reason why we get out of bed in the morning'. No matter how the word is translated, it is a significant tool that can be used to better understand yourself and how you can achieve individual wellbeing … and to live a longer, healthier and more present life.

To find our true Ikigai – or purpose – you need to reflect on what you love, what you are good at, what you can be paid for and what the world needs. This exercise needs to be done in complete honesty with oneself; otherwise the Ikigai, although found, might not lead to the profound happiness and wellbeing desired.

So, take pen and paper, sit down where you cannot be interrupted by others (or by your phone in particular) and write down:

A. Three things that you love
B. Three things you are good at
C. Three things you can be paid for
D. Three things you believe the world needs

Now, with the help of the diagram in Fig. 1.1, try to connect A and B to find your mission. Connect B and C to find your profession. Connect C and D to find your vocation. And finally, connect A and D to find your passion. Once you have these four categories, start thinking: What connects them? What is my Ikigai?

Influencing Your Wellbeing

Another secret shared by the citizens of Okinawa is best described by Viktor Frankl, the father of the school of psychotherapy based on finding meaning in life called logotherapy.

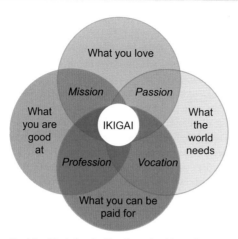

Fig. 1.1 Ikigai visualisation through a Venn diagram.

'Everything can be taken from a man but one thing: the last of the human freedoms – to choose one's attitude in any given set of circumstances, to choose one's one way.'

– FRANKL, 1962

There are many ways in which we can improve our wellbeing, and everyone should find and practise their own way of doing it. For instance, like the centenary Japanese people, we best keep a positive attitude towards the challenges life throws at us if we want to live longer and be less stressed. The latter is important, because a highly stressed, frenetic lifestyle has a degenerative effect on the cells of our bodies and it is linked to loss of memory, quicker ageing and lack of certain hormones, which can lead to depression (Joseph & Golden, 2017; Kiecolt-Glaser *et al.*, 2003). So, how do we keep stress to a manageable level and a positive attitude throughout?

Although as humans we tend to dwell on negatives because of our self-survival instinct that keeps us on the lookout for potential threats, complaining brings negativity into our life, especially when it's complaining about things we cannot control or change. Remember that our mindset is an immensely powerful tool and has a strong influence on our brain and how we perceive and deal with situations. Always try to think positively about what you are experiencing, celebrate every achievement, big or small, and face change and challenges with a cheerful outlook.

Secondly, many authors have studied change and its effect on people, and they have found that growth comes at the point of resistance; that being uncomfortable is the path to personal development and that from struggle come new skills (Stulberg & Magness, 2017). Change is scary, but change is the opposite of complacency. When everything is great and we are happy, we do not want to change; we become lazy. Sometimes a challenge is what we need to strive and grow. Even if you are in the optimal wellbeing state in most of its aspects, never stop challenging yourself to get out of the comfort zone, because change, whether it's a complete transformation or just a small adjustment, in addition to the acceptable dose of stress that comes with it, will improve your wellbeing. Furthermore, even if you end up failing, failure can be productive and give you an opportunity to analyse the problem from a different point of view.

So, find the courage to make change happen, to revitalise your brain with new challenges, to discover your Ikigai and to find your wellbeing!

And to maintain and improve your wellbeing, here is a list of other strategies you can use.

- Connect with other people: Socialising releases oxytocin and vasopressin, which are powerful antioxidants and anti-inflammatories, it improves your memory and it is also linked with a 50% increased likelihood of survival, hence a longer life (Brent *et al.*, 2014; García *et al.*, 2017; Holt-Lunstad *et al.*, 2010).

- Eat a healthy diet: A balanced diet can improve your energy levels, boost your immune system and reduce the risk of depression (Firth *et al.*, 2020).
- Be physically active: Regardless of the bout duration of exercise, physical activity decreases risks of diseases, anxiety and stress and improves mood, productivity and creativity (Anderson & Durstine, 2019; Jakicic *et al.*, 2019).
- Spend time in nature: Looking and being surrounded by nature increases vitality, autonomy, creativity and concentration and reduces overall stress (Capaldi *et al.*, 2015). Blue (water) and green (forest) areas are particularly good for resetting and relaxing.
- Give to others: Prosocial activities, charitable work and volunteering have been proven to increase your happiness, self-esteem and life satisfaction (Aknin *et al.*, 2020; Russell *et al.*, 2019).
- Practise mindfulness: Paying attention to the present moment through mindfulness and/ or meditation has been shown to improve physical performance and quality of sleep while reducing stress and anxiety. Additionally, it increases grey matter in the prefrontal cortex area, reducing cognitive decline (Jones *et al.*, 2020; Pernet *et al.*, 2021).
- Get enough sleep: It has been proven that adequate sleep is essential for consolidation and storing of new information, cognitive functioning and improved attention. Between 7 and 9 hours of sleep is the amount recommended to also reduce the risk of accident and injuries, and to improve overall mood and psychological wellbeing (Czeisler, 2011; Hirshkowitz *et al.*, 2015; Paruthi *et al.*, 2016).
- Plan holidays and time off work: Taking both short breaks and longer holidays during the year has been proven to decrease absenteeism, increase work engagement and reduce stress, among other benefits like increased quality of life and cognitive performance (Packer, 2021).
- Seek professional help if needed: When struggling with mental health issues or other health problems, seeking help from a qualified professional can be a crucial step towards improving your wellbeing (Jankowski *et al.*, 2020).

Due to the high physical and emotional demands of our job, we need to be cautious and learn how to manage our workload, balancing it with some of the recovery habits mentioned above, to reset our physical and mental state and be ready to help our patients.

This work-recovery equilibrium, dance even, is very subjective and can change throughout your life depending on your priorities and physical and mental state. But, by finding it, you could avoid what unfortunately can affect healthcare professionals who push themselves too much without recovering: burnout.

Burnout

Therapist burnout is the manifestation of both physical and mental stress that arises from being overworked or feeling undervalued within a work situation – or a lack of being challenged or being bored with one's current role. Burnout is included in the WHO's 11th Revision of the International Classification of Diseases (ICD-11) as an occupational phenomenon. It is not classified as a medical condition (WHO, 2022).

The WHO defines burnout as 'a syndrome conceptualised as resulting from chronic workplace stress that has not been successfully managed'. It is characterised by three dimensions (WHO, 2022):
- Feelings of energy depletion or exhaustion
- Increased mental distance from one's job, or feelings of negativism or cynicism related to one's job
- Reduced professional efficacy

Burnout refers specifically to phenomena in the occupational context and should not be applied to describe experiences in other areas of life. In 2020 the Chartered Society of Physiotherapy stated, 'People who experience burnout typically feel a mixture of symptoms that can be both physical and mental. Physical symptoms can manifest, such as chronic stress, headaches, and intestinal issues' (Blackburn & Mitchell, 2020). The end stage for those suffering from burnout is often a debilitating mental health condition such as clinical depression or anxiety. Burnout can also cause emotional exhaustion, leading to people feeling drained, unable to cope or focus and constantly tired. Performance at work is often affected, and the inability to separate work from home life can affect sleep patterns and the overall general health and wellbeing of a person.

This feeling of being overwhelmed or suffering from the stress of burnout as a physiotherapist has been described in several articles, including by Preece (2020), highlighting some of the symptoms of burnout, and Rodríguez-Nogueira *et al.* (2022), who concluded that higher levels of burnout resulted in lower levels of empathy amongst Spanish physiotherapists.

In professional- or elite-level sports, the physiotherapist can be working extended hours – sometimes alone – looking after the healthcare needs of the team or athlete that they are with and can be frequently challenged to take on roles that may sit outside of their professional scope of practice. The team physiotherapist can become the counsellor, medic and dispenser of medications – on top of their physiotherapy responsibilities. This can also be exacerbated by other tasks, including sorting out nutrition and hydration, checking into hotels and assisting with the kit. Here is a good example of where one loves the job, extra hours and so forth, so the balance is not 50/50.

In a Primary Care (UK National Health Service) setting, some physiotherapists work as First Contact Practitioners or Advanced Practitioners (FCPs or APs). The allotted appointment times can often be 15 or 20 minutes consistently throughout each day. The speed and number of patients that can attend clinics within a day or week can create the environment for an individual to feel burnt out or pressured to the point where they either need wellbeing support or consider changing their profession.

There is an assessment tool known as the Maslach Burnout Inventory (Maslach & Jackson, 1981) that, despite being some 40+ years old, can still be useful for today's clinician. The Maslach Burnout Inventory assesses an individual across five areas: emotional exhaustion, depersonalisation, personal accomplishment, cynicism and professional efficacy. It has subsequently been updated to include specific groups such as medical personnel and student groups.

So what can we do to avoid or reduce our potential for experiencing therapist burnout? It may sound simple, but taking care of ourselves through a good diet and maintaining a healthy exercise level is a good starting point. Take time away from the workplace – either with friends or family – and engage in activities that provide a diversion and interest to stimulate us.

It is important to be aware of the signs and symptoms of burnout at an early stage – this could be tiredness, reduction in concentration levels or recognising when our feelings of empathy towards our patients start to diminish. If one of the challenges is that it is difficult for us to recognise early signs of burnout, try to enlist the help of colleagues, friends and family. This may be a phenomenon we are able to recognise in our colleagues easier than we may be able to admit to ourselves.

The continual dilemma of 'living to work' or 'working to live' can drive people to push themselves beyond what they find acceptable or able to tolerate. This can often be the case at earlier stages of a physiotherapy career when you may be working hard to progress your career and not want to admit to a colleague or employer that you are struggling to cope with the demands upon you. One idea to help initiate conversations with colleagues and employers about the potential for burnout is the Mental Health UK 'Stress Bucket' worksheet (Mental Health UK, 2018). It can help to visualise stresses and consider ways of managing or reducing these stressors.

There are a number of other assessment tools that could help assess or develop our wellbeing. One such tool is the MTQ48, which is a validated measure for assessing mental toughness – or resilience (Clough *et al.*, 2002).

The components of mental toughness within this tool are illustrated in Fig. 1.2. The concept of mental toughness through the four 'C's can recognise positive and negative traits that can be developed to help an individual become more resilient to stress or personal challenge. This could help to improve the wellbeing of the physiotherapist and deal with adverse situations in a more capable way.

Resilience + Positivity = Mental Toughness

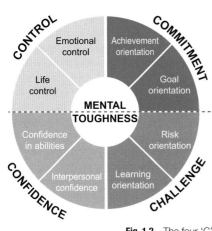

Resilience
The ability to recover from adversity

- Broadly explained by Control and Commitment
- Passive – it's a response
- Rearward looking – dealing with what has happened
- It helps you to survive

Positivity
The quality of having a positive attitude

- Broadly explained by Challenge and Confidence
- Active – it's an optimistic anticipation
- Forward looking – dealing with now and what's ahead
- It helps you to thrive

Fig. 1.2 The four 'C's. (Courtesy D. Strycharczyk.)

Mental and physical wellbeing is the bedrock on which our caring profession has its foundations, and we should look out for ourselves and our colleagues to maintain a healthy and supportive environment for all.

Nozedar & O'Shea (2023) published a report on the prevalence of burnout in first-contact physiotherapists working in primary care. They found that 13% of those who responded were suffering from burnout, with a further 16% at risk of burnout. The shocking statistic of 78% of respondents were either exhausted or at risk of exhaustion. 'The results from this study show that 10+ hours of non-clinical time per month significantly reduces burnout when compared to 2 hours or less per month and highlights a positive trend in that the more non-clinical time per month the lower the burnout score of that individual.'

Five Key Takeaways

1. Remember that you can only truly have the energy and enthusiasm towards those you work with as patients by ensuring that you take the care and attention to look after yourself first.
2. Understand what contributes to burnout and influences your wellbeing.
3. The Japanese concept of Ikigai can be a useful tool for improving individual wellbeing. It requires honest reflection on what one loves, what one is good at, what one can be paid for and what the world needs.
4. Regular self-assessment and peer discussion can help in early identification and prevention of burnout. It's important to create a supportive work environment where employees feel comfortable discussing their mental health and burnout symptoms.
5. Maintaining wellbeing in a demanding profession such as physiotherapy involves a combination of strategies like keeping a positive mindset, embracing change and challenges, maintaining social connections, practising mindfulness, maintaining physical health and seeking professional help when needed.

Five Self-Directed Reflections

1. Are there any signs of burnout you may have overlooked in your current professional situation? If so, what measures can you take to address them?

2. Reflect on the balance between your work and personal life. How can you ensure a healthier balance to reduce potential burnout?
3. How can you incorporate tools like the Maslach Burnout Inventory or the MTQ48 into your routine to monitor your mental health and resilience?
4. What are the key components of your own Ikigai, and how do they intersect to form your purpose?
5. Reflect on a recent stressful situation. How did you respond to it, and how might you apply the same wellbeing strategies suggested in this chapter to similar situations in the future?

References

Aknin, L., Dunn, E., Proulx, J., Lok, I., & Norton, M. (2020). Does spending money on others promote happiness? A registered replication report. *Journal of Personality and Social Psychology, 119*(2), e15.

Anderson, E., & Durstine, J. (2019). Physical activity, exercise, and chronic diseases: A brief review. *Sports Medicine and Health Science, 1*(1), 3–10.

Blackburn, J., & Mitchell, J. (2020). Physio burnout. *CSP Frontline, 9*, 20–21.

Brent, L. J., Chang, S., Gariépy, J., & Platt, M. (2014). The neuroethology of friendship. *Annals of the New York Academy of Sciences, 1316*(1), 1–17.

Capaldi, C., Passmore, H., Nisbet, E., Zelenski, J., & Dopko, R. (2015). Flourishing in nature: A review of the benefits of connecting with nature and its application as a wellbeing intervention. *International Journal of Wellbeing, 5*(4), 1–16.

Clough, P., Earle, K., & Sewell, D. (2002). Mental toughness: The concept and its measurement. In I. Cockerill (Ed.), *Solutions in Sport Psychology* (pp. 32–43). London: Thomson.

Czeisler, C. A. (2011). Impact of sleepiness and sleep deficiency on public health – utility of biomarkers. *Journal of Clinical Sleep Medicine, 7*(5 Suppl), S6–S8.

Firth, J., Gangwisch, J., Borsini, A., Wootton, R., & Mayer, E. (2020). Food and mood: How do diet and nutrition affect mental wellbeing? *BMJ, 369*, 1–4.

Frankl, V. E. (1962). *Man's search for meaning: An introduction to logotherapy.* Boston, MA: Beacon Press.

García, H., Miralles, F., & Cleary, H. (2017). *Ikigai: The Japanese secret to a long and happy life.* New York: Penguin Books.

Gavrilova, N. S., & Gavrilov, L. (2012). Comments on dietary restriction, Okinawa diet and longevity. *Gerontology, 58*, 221–223.

Hirshkowitz, M., Whiton, K., Albert, S., Alessi, C., Bruni, O., & DonCarlos, L. (2015). National Sleep Foundation's sleep time duration recommendations: Methodology and results summary. *Sleep Health, 1*, 40–43.

Holt-Lunstad, J., Smith, T., & Layton, J. (2010). Social relationships and mortality risk: A meta-analytic review. *PLoS Medicine, 7*(7), 1–20.

Huberman Lab Podcast. (2022). Science-based tools for increasing happiness. Podcast 98, 14 November. YouTube. Available at https://www.youtube.com/watch?v=LTGGyQS1fZE.

Jakicic, J., Kraus, W., Powell, K., Campbell, W., Janz, K., Troiano, R., Sprow, K., Torres, A., & Piercy, K. (2019). Association between bout duration of physical activity and health: Systematic review. *Medicine and Science in Sports and Exercise, 51*(6), 1213–1219.

Jankowski, P., Sandage, S., Bell, C., Davis, D., Porter, E., Jessen, M., Motzny, C., Ross, K., & Owen, J. (2020). Virtue, flourishing, and positive psychology in psychotherapy: An overview and research prospectus. *Psychotherapy, 57*(3), 291.

Jones, B. J., Kaur, S., Miller, M., & Spencer, R. (2020). Mindfulness-based stress reduction benefits psychological well-being, sleep quality, and athletic performance in female collegiate rowers. *Frontiers in Psychology, 11*, 1–10.

Joseph, J., & Golden, S. (2017). Cortisol dysregulation: The bidirectional link between stress, depression, and type 2 diabetes mellitus. *Annals of the New York Academy of Science, 1391*(1), 20–34.

Kiecolt-Glaser, J., Preacher, K., MacCallum, R., Atkinson, C., Malarkey, W., & Glaser, R. (2003). Chronic stress and age-related increases in the proinflammatory cytokine IL-6. *Proceedings of the National Academy of Sciences, 100*(15), 9090–9095.

La Placa, V., McNaught, A., & Knight, A. (2013). Discourse on wellbeing in research and practice. *International Journal of Wellbeing, 3*(1), 116–125.

Lawton, M. (1983). The varieties of wellbeing. *Experimental Aging Research, 9*(2), 65–72.

Knight, A., & McNaught, A. (2011). *Understanding wellbeing: An introduction for students and practitioners of health and social care.* Banbury: Lantern Publishing.

Maslach, C., & Jackson, S. E. (1981). The measurement of experienced burnout. *Journal of Organizational Behavior, 2*(2), 99–113. https://doi.org/10.1002/job.403002020.

Mental Health UK. (2018). The Stress Bucket. Available at https://mentalhealth-uk.org/blog/the-stress-bucket/.

Nozedar, L., & O'Shea, S (2023). What is the prevalence of burnout amongst first contact physiotherapists working within primary care? *Musculoskeletal Care*, 1–10. https://doi.org/10.1002/msc.1752.

Packer, J. (2021). Taking a break: Exploring the restorative benefits of short breaks and vacations. *Annals of Tourism Research Empirical Insights, 2*(1), 100006.

Paruthi, S., Brooks, L., D'Ambrosio, C., Hall, W., Kotagal, S., Lloyd, R., Malow, B., Maski, K., Nichols, C., Quan, S., Rosen, C., Troester, M., & Wise, M (2016). Consensus statement of the American Academy of Sleep Medicine on the recommended amount of sleep for healthy children: Methodology and discussion. *Journal of Clinical Sleep Medicine, 12*(11), 1549–1561.

Pernet, C. R., Belov, N., Delorme, A., & Zammit, A. (2021). Mindfulness related changes in grey matter: A systematic review and meta-analysis. *Brain Imaging and Behaviour, 15*, 2720–2730.

Preece, C. (2020). Stress and burnout in physiotherapists: A literature review of causative factors, the impact on patient care, and coping strategies. *Physiotherapy, 107*(S1), e81–e82. https://doi.org/10.1016/j.physio.2020.03.112.

Rodríguez-Nogueira, Ó., Leirós-Rodríguez, R., Pinto-Carral, A., Álvarez-Álvarez, M. J., Fernández-Martínez, E., & Moreno-Poyato, A. R. (2022). The relationship between burnout and empathy in physiotherapists: A cross-sectional study. *Annals of medicine, 54*(1), 933–940. https://doi.org/10.1080/07853890.2022.2059102.

Russell, A., Nyame-Mensah, A., de Wit, A., & Handy, F. (2019). Volunteering and wellbeing among ageing adults: A longitudinal analysis. *VOLUNTAS: International Journal of Voluntary and Nonprofit Organizations, 30*, 115–128.

Stulberg, B., & Magness, S. (2017). *Peak performance: Elevate your game, avoid burnout, and thrive with the new science of success.* Emmaus, PA: Rodale Books.

Willcox, B., Willcox, D., Todoroki, H., Fujiyoshi, A., Yano, K., He, Q., Curb, J., & Suzuki, M. (2007). Caloric restriction, the traditional Okinawan diet, and healthy ageing: The diet of the world's longest-lived people and its potential impact on morbidity and life span. *Annals of the New York Academy of Sciences, 1114*, 434–455.

Willcox, D., Scapagnini, G., & Wilcox, B. (2014). Healthy ageing diets other than the Mediterranean: A focus on the Okinawan diet. *Mechanisms of Ageing and Development.* 136–137, 148–162.

World Health Organization. (2022). International Classification of Diseases (ICD) revision 11. Available at https://icd.who.int/en.

Further Reading

García, H., Miralles, F., & Cleary, H. (2017). *Ikigai: The Japanese secret to a long and happy life.* New York: Penguin Books.

Nozedar, L., & O'Shea, S. (2023). What is the prevalence of burnout amongst first contact physiotherapists working within primary care? *Musculoskeletal Care, 21*(3), 776–785. https://doi.org/10.1002/msc.1752.

Sinek, S. (2011). *Start with why.* London: Penguin Books.

Strycharczyk, D., Clough, P., & Perry, J. (2021). *Developing mental toughness: Strategies to improve performance, resilience and wellbeing in individuals and organizations* (ed 3). London: Kogan Page.

TEDx. How to build your well-being to thrive – Dr Beth Cabrera [Video]. YouTube.

CHAPTER 2

Purpose and Values

Emmanuel Ovola ▦ Ana Mali

'Passion for your work is a little bit of discovery, followed by a lot of development, and then a lifetime of deepening.'
Angela Duckworth, psychologist and thought leader on 'Grit', 2016

Introduction

Identifying the core values that motivate us each morning is crucial for sustained wellbeing, achievement and high performance.

High achievers are often characterised by their discipline, goal-oriented mindset, consistent schedules and a lean towards perfectionism. Their actions and aspirations are deeply rooted in a clearly defined purpose and set of values, steering both their personal and professional journeys.

The values that play such an important part in steering their lives are mostly born out of life experiences. They act as principles which guide everyday behaviours, help enhance self-awareness and provide a personal perspective. We have all experienced moments and situations that have likely shaped our values from an early age. In this chapter we will dive into how these values, these guiding principles, can create and enhance success in our personal and professional lives.

What Is Purpose?

Why do we do what we do? Why do we act in certain ways? Mostly, we are guided by our purpose and values. Specifically, purpose is the underlying 'why' behind how we act. It is the fuel to our fire. When we resonate with our actions it is likely because we are in alignment with our purpose. It's the underlying force that propels us forward, the compelling reason that stirs us from bed each morning, eager to embrace the day ahead.

Purpose transcends professional and personal domains. It is the driving force behind any development plan, and as mentioned, it is a key factor in determining success in your career. Professionally, purpose helps to define career objectives, providing a sense of direction and motivation. By having a clear purpose, individuals are more likely to stay focused on their long-term goals and can also use it to measure progress and success. It can be used as a tool to help individuals to reflect on their skills and strengths and identify areas for improvement, aspects vital to incremental improvement.

At a personal level, purpose can provide a sense of meaning and fulfilment in life. As the old saying goes, it is the life you have lived in your years, not the number of years you have lived in your life. Purpose can be used to help individuals to identify their passions and interests and determine how they can use their skills and interests to make a positive contribution to their lives and the lives of others. It can also be used to develop resilience and to help individuals to cope with difficult times. Having a clear grasp of purpose can help to provide direction and focus and can help individuals to develop both professionally and personally. Understanding and aligning with one's purpose is the key to leading a fulfilling and successful life.

How to Use Purpose in Physiotherapy for Professional and Personal Development

Physiotherapy is a vital healthcare profession that aims to help people improve and achieve their highest holistic wellbeing, thereby improving quality of life and benefiting their families and caregivers. There are numerous specialisations in physiotherapy, including musculoskeletal, neurological, paediatric, community-based, sports and others, which all carry equal importance. Each specialisation is constantly improving and evolving due to advances in high-quality scientific research, underscoring the importance of physiotherapy and its potential for increasing its accessibility and functionality in the future.

Continuous professional development of services and practitioners is crucial to providing reliable and high-quality services. The strengths of physiotherapists lie in their proficiency with anatomy, physiology and other science- and health-related areas such as health and physical activity promotion, injury prevention, rehabilitation and the management of various injuries and physical conditions. The enduring goal is always to improve the client's physical, psychological, emotional and social wellbeing (World Physiotherapy, n.d.).

The purpose of physiotherapy for professional development is to create and develop treatment plans tailored to the individual patient's needs and provide the highest level of care possible. It is essential to make work more effective and improve client outcomes. An investment in professional development can result in economic benefits. Therefore, each year, reviewing and re-evaluating goals and aiming to further improve is necessary. This commitment to professional development can ensure physiotherapists continue to develop skills and knowledge while following and keeping up with the latest guidelines, which enables them to stay up to date with the latest advances in the field and provide the best possible care.

Furthermore, a physiotherapist should always find purpose in improving soft skills and prioritise their application in their physiotherapy practice. The purpose of learning and using emotional intelligence; professional, respectful and transparent communication; and active listening is to create positive relationships with patients/clients, their families or caregivers and colleagues. Building solid relationships, trust and rapport is possible with these skills.

To illustrate this, let us consider a scenario where you visit a doctor or healthcare professional with a busy work schedule and the communication starts roughly from their side. How did you respond to that? Did you feel shocked and more likely to respond to them with the same tone and attitude? Even though the appointment was concluded and solved, the added stress created by the interactions may affect both parties negatively. Unfortunately, this scenario may happen too often.

Instead, a positive attitude, empathy, nonverbal communication cues and finding common ground can change the direction of an appointment/conversation and create an effective collaborative environment.

The reason to become a better professional is for the clients: firstly, past clients who have highlighted areas in which physiotherapists needed to improve their knowledge and skills or search for additional support to provide other perspectives and advice if required; the second reason is that physiotherapists working with clients daily may present new challenges requiring continual growth and learning. Finally, many clients or patients are thankful for the physiotherapist's work in regaining their functionality and quality of life, allowing them to reach their potential – clients who got a chance to regain and re-evaluate their purpose.

By having a purpose and aiming to improve professionally in physiotherapy, health professionals can experience development personally and professionally. The latter benefits both professionals and also their clients. In addition, by becoming a physiotherapist, professionals can focus their energy and attention on activities that promote growth and success, allowing them to set clear and achievable goals and stay focused and motivated. To attain personal development and determine how to improve, it is crucial to ask for and accept feedback and constructive criticism from approachable and trustworthy individuals, such as close friends, family members or colleagues.

A Reflection From Manni on Purpose

Grow proud of what and who you become through the years. It can be challenging sometimes to be proud of what you do and how you live – but the key is to reflect. Once you know where you have been, it provides you with the context of where you may want to go; without this understanding, you may not know what you are seeking in life or what you need. The final destination is important, sure – but the big thing is how motivated you are to get there. Can you weather the storms? Do you understand the path today, to get to where you need to be? The why, what and how of today are key. We all can and will create a special life, provided we identify and know our direction. It's like trying to walk or drive without the GPS on … it is pointless.

Purpose Then Mastery, or Mastery Then Purpose?

Let's consider a broader perspective of purpose. It is important to examine opposite views to the long-heralded advice that you should simply 'follow your passion' in life. Renowned author, deep work productivity expert and Georgetown University tenured professor Cal Newport describes an intriguing counterpoint in his book 'So Good They Can't Ignore You' and upcoming book 'Deep Life'. He suggests that advice to find your passion or purpose and follow it can be misleading and, ultimately, detrimental.

Cal has a provocative view in which he proposes that we should go wide and explore a range of experiences before committing to what we truly deem as our purpose. How you end up loving what you do as a living, he suggests, is more about getting very good at an endeavour, and the passion for that path will follow. Mastery therefore is the key to unearthing your purpose.

Consider an amateur baker who is devoted to baking; just because they love the act does not mean they will love creating shelves full of cakes or breads for a bakery, creating advertising to promote their store and even running the accounts of a small business. For them, a career as a baker could be a painful one, despite it seemingly aligning with their passion. They may find little enjoyment in such a career path … and this distinction is crucial. We must acknowledge that we are not hardwired for a single vocation, and our interests can evolve over time.

The critical takeaway here is not to devalue purpose. Instead, it is to understand that not loving every aspect of your job when you are a beginner does not mean that it cannot grow to become your passion or purpose. It is important to experiment and gain experience in many avenues. This exposure to new stimuli and continued learning will gradually guide your career path. As you get better and achieve mastery a love and passion may follow.

Align your work with your values. Do not fixate on landing the perfect role or job immediately. Step out of your comfort zone, take note of what resonates with you, experience failures, celebrate victories and learn from it all. That is most important.

Conduct a small experiment with your colleagues, mentors or people you admire. Ask them about their journey to their current position. No doubt, you will find that some attribute their career path to serendipity or to pure unconscious luck or chance. They did not intentionally end up where they are. They did not carefully plan the road. It simply happened. But now they feel it is their purpose.

Use this insight to gain confidence in your flexibility. As you develop expertise in areas that are both rare and valuable, you will start to differentiate yourself. As an entrepreneur and digital creator Dan Koe and famed comic strip writer Scott Adams (he of Dilbert Fame) suggest, layer your personal strengths, skills and experiences to create a truly unique proposition. This is when your purpose becomes clear. This is when you become genuinely valuable and unique, aligning your identity with your experiences – and, ultimately, unearthing your true purpose.

Values

Self-awareness and reflection are core teachings in physiotherapy courses worldwide. They impart models, frameworks and processes to students to deepen their understanding of clinical experiences. But have you considered the driving force behind why these experiences happen – your values? Figuring out what your values are and ultimately who you are, despite its tribulations, is the most rewarding work that you can do.

Who are you … really? Consider this question for a moment. Would you be able to answer it well?

Too often, when asked 'Who are you?', we reply with our name, job title and perhaps for a bit of flavour where we are from – 'I'm Ana, I'm a physiotherapist from Slovenia' – but how much does this statement truly convey who we really are? For all we know there could be 500 physiotherapists called Ana from Slovenia. Yet none of us are the same; as humans we are all unique, and we must be able to articulate and show this. Our individualities differentiate us … and act as our superpowers.

To authentically represent ourselves we must go beyond surface-level descriptors, like job titles and origins. We must bring this authenticity to our interactions and to our day-to-day experiences. While the following may sound slightly abstract, think of yourself as a diamond for a moment. Like diamonds, each of us is one of a kind, with no two alike. Formed under tremendous heat and pressure, over a timeline of millions of years, diamonds have a specific arrangement of atoms and inclusions that give them a distinct fingerprint, making each one truly unique. Similarly, our life experiences, beliefs and values shape our individuality, setting us apart from everyone else. So, when we answer 'who we are' with surface-level descriptors, not only are we doing ourselves a major injustice, but we are also limiting the potential to develop meaningful relationships with others.

Much like how a diamond's beauty is revealed through careful cutting and polishing, the intellectual and self-reflective process to understand our values and purpose can reveal our authentic selves, our distinct fingerprint. This journey of self-discovery allows us to embrace our individuality, directing us towards a more successful and fulfilling life.

Unfortunately, in modern times, we are often not the ones behind the wheel for this journey. External influences tend to shape our experiences and direct our lives – influences like social media. We avoid the hard work of learning about our fears, frustrations and energisers; instead we allow our lives to be defined by others and what society wants and demands of us.

As described in the journal *Behavioural Sciences,* values are the fundamental beliefs and behaviours that a person holds in his or her life (Gamage *et al.*, 2021). They shape the enduring feelings

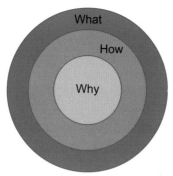

Fig. 2.1 Golden Circle. (*Courtesy* Simon Sinek. Available at https://simonsinek.com/golden-circle/. Accessed 11 March 2024.)

and attitudes that we attain through our genetics and our lived experiences from a young age. Put simply, they are the filters through which we interpret the world and therefore guide our everyday behaviour (Urbany *et al.*, 2008).

Values are the measuring stick by which we determine how we think and what we do. They are the guiding principles that define how we act when nobody else is watching. They are reflected in the way we behave each and every day and are often expressed as single words, such as honesty, loyalty, dedication or caring, or sometimes as short sentences.

Dr Michael Gervais, a renowned performance psychologist who has worked with the Super Bowl–winning Seattle Seahawks, notes that our values are 'guiding principles' that serve to align our thoughts, words and actions. If we fail to live by our values it may result in a life shaped by others' perceptions, and one in which we never find balance or fulfilment (Clancy & Dunne, 2022, 33:05).

Leadership expert Simon Sinek crafted the Golden Circle (Fig. 2.1) concept to illustrate the significance of values in relation to how we behave. Starting at the centre of the circle is 'Why', representing our core values and beliefs, surrounded by 'How' and 'What', symbolising our actions and the result of our actions, respectively. By understanding and embracing our values, we can create a strong foundation for our purpose, navigating our careers and lives with clarity and conviction (Sinek, 2009).

Think of values as fully independent decision guides that allow us to feel comfortable with specific behaviours or feel resistance towards others. Each moment of the day, whether we realise it or not, we are deciding how to spend our time, what we pay attention to and where we should direct our energy. Right now, you are choosing to read this book, maybe because continuous improvement or ambition is a value you hold. There are infinite things you could be doing but you chose to be here, and this in and of itself is your value system working for you.

Personal and Professional Values

Personal values, however, are not alone. Professional values exist and are often seen printed on email headers or on clinic walls or spoken about in organisational communications. While these values may differ from our personal ones, the origin and role of these guides remain the same – to create coherence and consistency in how we (as employees or stakeholders) behave within and as a part of the organisation.

Gorenak and Košir (2012) emphasise the significance of organisational values as the core principles and beliefs fundamental to an organisation's existence. These values shape the culture, influence employee engagement, and guide management and staff in achieving the organisation's mission. They are the basic ingredients of the organisation's recipe. During onboarding, management teams share and impart these values to new joining employees, in the hope that the employee will uphold these principles throughout their employment.

The American Physical Therapy Association (2021) posits seven core values that represent the physical therapy and physiotherapy profession: accountability, altruism, compassion, caring, excellence, integrity and professional duty.

A study on 14 practising and experienced physiotherapists in Australia found a wide but overlapping trend in their professional values. It showed the alignment of physiotherapists with our purported professional values and the variances of personal values within our profession. For the study, Aguilar *et al.* (2012) defined a professional value 'as a principle or standard that an individual perceives as important to their professional role'. A prominent example of a value was 'making a difference to updating skills', and all values fell within three themes: 'the patient and the patient-therapist partnership', 'physiotherapy knowledge skills and practice' and finally 'altruistic values'. The study highlights that while there is diversity in our values, certain themes exist and direct physiotherapists in this shared profession. Varying professional roles may lead us to encounter a wide array of values. What we must consider and aim for is how we can, firstly, identify the organisation's professional values and what our interpretation of those values are and, secondly, how we can aim to live these values in our day-to-day interactions and behaviours as part of the organisation.

Learning what your organisational values are is an extremely worthwhile exercise. It can help you align with the overall purpose of the group and enhance your happiness and connection to your role. If you are your organisation, consider how you communicate and embody your values with your clients or customers.

So, as discussed, personal and professional values may intertwine but are not always carbon copies. Personal values evolve from our backgrounds, encounters and convictions, while professional values stem from industry norms, ethical guidelines and workplace demands. Ideally, syncing personal and professional values generates harmony and coherence in our actions. However, divergence may cause inner turmoil, waning job contentment and potential moral difficulties.

This turmoil can particularly manifest in employment. Imagine Laura. She's a highly skilled and recently graduated physiotherapist. Laura has begun a new role at a local but high-profile physiotherapy clinic.

Laura, being very self-aware, understands that her values are and always have been about compassion, holistic care and providing patient autonomy. These aren't just words to her – they're her guiding principles; they shape her approach to care. For Laura, care is comprehensive. It's patient centred. It's personal.

Then comes the hard bit: the clinic Laura's joined. They do things differently. Their values are all about efficiency, number of visits per patient and rapid new patient acquisition. It's a business model, and the bottom line is profitability. For them, it's simple: get people signed up for sessions and keep them in the loop. And do it all fast. Long-term health and autonomy? They often take a back seat.

For Laura, this is a challenge. A big one. Her personal commitment to holistic care, to patient empowerment? It's clashing with the clinic's drive for speed, for turnover. Laura's feeling the pressure. She's rushing her treatments. Making decisions that, deep down, she knows might not be best for her patients in the long run.

Take this one case: a tennis player with a recurring shoulder injury. Laura thinks a comprehensive, patient-centred rehabilitation plan is best. But the clinic? They want passive treatments as the main approach. Laura goes along with it. But just as she feared, the player becomes reliant on the sessions and displays an increased sense of reliance on the treatments. The patient's self-efficacy is dwindling.

Laura's story? It's a wake-up call. A reminder of what can happen when personal and professional values don't line up. Laura's job satisfaction? It's plummeting. She's even questioning her career choice. That's how important it is to get personal and professional values on the same page.

In the end, Laura makes a move. She leaves the clinic. She joins a practice that's all about holistic, patient-centred care. It's a better fit for her personal values. And guess what? Her job satisfaction skyrockets. She's providing the kind of care she truly believes in. The kind of care her patients deserve.

Connecting With Others Through Purpose and Values

'*You are the average of the five people you spend the most time with.*'

– JIM ROHN (1930–2009), ENTREPRENEUR, AUTHOR AND MOTIVATIONAL SPEAKER

It should be no surprise to learn that who we surround ourselves with is of vital importance. You may have heard of the above idea that we are the average of the five people we encounter most. While the evidence and sentiment of this are debated amongst behavioural scientists and psychologists, we need to focus on and appreciate why we have connected with these five individuals. There are clues as to who we are as people in there.

Being social creatures, humans crave connection, seeking tribes to strive and thrive together. It is an innate desire embedded in our DNA. But how do we choose who joins us on life's journey and who deserves our time?

Our values hold the key to these choices. Shared values facilitate bonds with like-minded people who echo our beliefs and ideals. These ties have a profound impact on personal growth, swaying our perceptions, attitudes and convictions about relationships and the world at large.

When we align with people with similar values, we establish a supportive network, nurturing mutual understanding and compassion. These relationships deepen, as trust and relatedness flourish when our core values align. Our surrounding environment tends to blossom when we can genuinely express our thoughts, emotions and beliefs without fearing judgement, or when we can stay true to our personal values despite how what we say or do may be received.

Being around these like-minded individuals can fuel motivation and inspiration. Observing peers chase passions and embody similar values to ours can in turn inspire us to follow suit. This encouragement spurs us to chase our own aspirations more vigorously, meaning heightened fulfilment in our careers and lives. Consequently, connection with others that hold vastly different values may invite conflict and confusion within the relationships. If we perceive others to be acting against our guiding principles, bonds can become broken and it can even harm our mental and emotional wellbeing.

By seeking connections with value-aligned individuals, we foster a nurturing atmosphere that bolsters personal growth, deepens bonds and enriches our lives. To maximise our relationships and life journey, it is crucial to remain mindful of our values and connect with those who resonate with our core beliefs or, at the very least, who can respect and acknowledge our core beliefs.

Defining Your Values

Many formats and processes are suggested to identify and determine our core values. A particularly effective way is by defining a list of anti-values. *Anti-values* are the behaviours, intentions and actions that frustrate us even to think about. They are the actions that make us feel regret and irritate us if we see others doing them. We can use these irritations to learn who we are not and use this as a guiding path to learning who we are. Later in the chapter we will share key actions to do this.

Another method to locate and define your values is by creating your flock of values, your 'black sheep values', as Brant Menswar, author of 'Black Sheep', says (Menswar, 2020). These are your non-negotiables. Start with going through a values list and circling the words that resonate with you, such as empathy, faith, integrity, fairness, determination, courage, resilience, compassion, optimism, authenticity, curiosity, success, trust and connection. That might bring you to 30 values that you gravitate to.

Go back through your list, grouping the words by likeness. For example, 'empathy' and 'sympathy' can go in one box, and 'success' and 'aspiration' in another. When you have created a subset of five boxes of words that are similar, pick the word from each box that speaks to you in your heart, head and gut. This is your initial flock of five black sheep values. The next step is critical. They need to live and breathe. They need to be you, your unique fingerprint of values, as it were. Track your daily actions and evaluate when these values show up, how frequently and how pronounced and obvious. You will notice them daily. One or two values may change with time, but for the most part they are yours to stay for a long time.

Behaviours, Values and Soft Skills

In physiotherapy, values include soft skills and behaviours that foster an environment promoting wellbeing, trust and progress. Physiotherapists are positioned to play a leading role as providers whose priority is delivering value-based care (Cook *et al.*, 2021). Solid and robust relationships can be built by understanding and comprehending clients' or patients' unique goals and requirements. Values such as friendship, respect, safety and security are sometimes subconsciously created. Alongside effective communication, collaboration and patient-centred care, achieving one's full potential is possible.

When clients feel respected, understood and valued, they are more likely to follow treatment plans, seek assistance and report issues and injuries more frequently. Additionally, possessing emotional intelligence and stress management helps physiotherapists to identify, support and manage their own and others' emotions and stress levels. As a result, they can respond adequately, offer better support and reduce the risk of burnout and injury.

Moreover, being open-minded, showing compassion and empathy, and considering clients' values and beliefs make physiotherapists more adaptable and practical when working with clients of diverse backgrounds, cultures and values. Furthermore, physiotherapists should see their work environment as supportive; if their supervisor or manager does not present similar values, they will usually consider changing their place of employment.

The value of professional development in physiotherapy and maintaining a high level of professionalism focuses on effective communication, evaluating situations subjectively and objectively, demonstrating ethical behaviour and respecting boundaries, all of which promote a positive reputation for the profession. Additionally, taking responsibility for meeting commitments, providing support, being responsible for one's own actions and being accountable are values that can only contribute to personal and professional growth. Commitment, passion, a strong work ethic, positive attitudes, a positive mindset, completing tasks on time, integrity and motivation and interaction with peers can bring a good reputation at work, respect and personal satisfaction. Moreover, developing and building leadership skills can help physiotherapists guide their team towards progress and be productive without constant supervision.

James Clear, author of the excellent 'Atomic Habits', expertly summarises the link between behaviour and identity when he notes that 'every action you take is a vote for the type of person you wish to become'; we would argue that you are also voting for the type of person you wish to be, right here and now (Clear, 2018).

Purpose and Values in Physiotherapy – Bringing This to Life

'An enduring belief that a specific mode of conduct or end-state of existence is personally or socially preferable to an opposite or converse mode of conduct or end-state of existence.'

– MILTON ROKEACH (1973)

Defining values can be extremely important in the way physiotherapists approach their life and career. This frames how we treat others everywhere.

An example of this is the way we approach patients with certain religious beliefs. How do we support them to develop? How do we create an environment for patients to feel comfortable? Muslim women will at times prefer to see female physiotherapists, so we need to ensure we value this preference. We build that through having a form prior to attendance, asking what the preference of care is. This can create a better experience for the patients. It can reduce anxiety and support a fluid and smooth attendance to access services. This will then tie into the purpose as you navigate your purpose as a physiotherapist.

It is never too late for us to review the purpose in our profession, and if anything, it can be continuous. We will always refine the way we interact with patients and do our job. It is essentially how we can mould and shape the life we live and how this feeds into the profession. The purpose and values go hand in hand to create a more in-depth perspective.

Five Key Takeaways

1. Our values align with who we are now. They drive our behaviours both personally and professionally.
2. Understand that your values will evolve over time. Create time and space so that you can re-evaluate your purpose.
3. Finding out what they are and aligning them to our purpose is one of the most rewarding things we can do. It is also a key ingredient to a successful and fulfilled career.
4. Physiotherapy can create solid and robust relationships and offer patient-centred care based on values.
5. Each year, reassess and re-evaluate your purpose and values alongside your goals and beliefs. If you do not create a purpose someone will assign you one.

Five Self-Directed Reflections

1. It is important to reflect on why you value what you do, on a consistent basis.
2. Think about how this will affect the way you work – and what you need from your career.
3. Every day can guide you to where you need to be; build in ways to evaluate your progress and path on a daily basis.
4. Reflect with people around you and create a healthy environment to discuss and build trust.
5. Show interest in things you do not know, creating moments to learn more which add to your lived experience.

References

Aguilar, A., Stupans, I., Scutter, S., & King, S. (2012). Exploring professionalism: The professional values of Australian occupational therapists. *Australian Occupational Therapy Journal, 59*(3), 209–217.

American Physical Therapy Association. (2021). Core values for the physical therapist and physical therapist assistant. Available at https://www.apta.org/apta-and-you/leadership-and-governance/policies/core-values-for-the-physical-therapist-and-physical-therapist-assistant. Accessed 16 May 2023.

Clancy, D., & Dunne, C. (Hosts). (2022). *#164 Dr Michael Gervais (164)* [Audio Podcast Episode]. In *Sleep Eat Perform Repeat*. Hauora. Available at https://sleepeatperformrepeat.com/164-dr-michael-gervais.

Clear, J. (2018). *Atomic habits: The life-changing million-copy# 1 bestseller.* New York, NY: Random House.

Cook, C., Denninger, T., Lewis, J., Diener, I., & Thigpen, C. (2021). Providing value-based care as a physiotherapist. *Archives of Physiotherapy, 11*(12). https://doi.org/10.1186/s40945-021-00107-0.

Duckworth, A. (2016). *Grit: The power of passion and perseverance.* New York, NY: Scribner/Simon & Schuster.

Gamage, K. A. A., Dehideniya, D. M. S. C. P. K., & Ekanayake, S. Y. (2021). The role of personal values in learning approaches and student achievements. *Behavioral Sciences, 11*(7), 102. https://doi.org/10.3390/bs11070102.

Gorenak, M. & Košir, S. (2012). The importance of organizational values for organization. Knowledge and Learning: Global Empowerment; Proceedings of the Management, Knowledge and Learning International Conference 2012. International School for Social and Business Studies, Celje, Slovenia.

Menswar, B. (2020). *Black sheep: Unleash the extraordinary, awe-inspiring, undiscovered you.* Vancouver: Page Two Books.

Rokeach, M. (1973). *The nature of human values.* New York: The Free Press.

Sinek, S. (2009). *Start with why: How great leaders inspire everyone to take action.* New York: Portfolio.

Urbany, J. E., Reynolds, T. J., & Phillips, J. M. (2008). How to make values count in everyday decisions. *MIT Sloan Management Review.* Available at https://sloanreview.mit.edu/article/how-to-make-values-count-in-everyday-decisions/. Accessed 16 May 2023.

World Physiotherapy. (n.d.). What is physiotherapy? Available at https://world.physio/resources/what-is-physiotherapy.

CHAPTER 3

Habits – Sleep, Nutrition and Recovery

Paul Stevens ■ Matthew Bruno

'The only comparison I should be making is with myself. Will I be better tomorrow than I am today? Will I be more thoughtful, more intentional, more purposeful in the future than I am right now? Do my habits, routines, rituals and actions match my intention to be better tomorrow than I am today? These questions are the gateway to excellence because living a life of excellence is about the fanatical pursuit of gradual improvement.'

– Ryan Hawk, best-selling author and host of *The Learning Leader Show* podcast, 2022

CHAPTER OUTLINE

Introduction

Habits are autonomous, repeated actions and behaviours that we employ every day, for different outcomes or purposes. They may be performed out of necessity or survival, to produce a particular outcome or event, or even as a specific emotional or physical response. It is often felt that our success in each facet of life is a collective result of both positive and negative habits. These practices are often developed because of the way we wish to live our lives, and we learn them from an early age. For example, brushing your teeth before you go to bed, exercising at predetermined times at school or eating your vegetables with dinner are simple, common things that are ingrained into our daily routine to ensure we live a healthy lifestyle.

Just as we develop habits with positive effects in mind, we can just as easily create bad habits that impact our ability to thrive in our environment or context. Smoking, drinking alcohol and living a sedentary life are recognised as unhealthy habits and all have well-documented ill effects on our health. Eating meals irregularly or not at all, working for free outside of rostered hours and spending copious amounts of time on social media before going to bed can all be bad habits that we likely perform more often than we will admit, without truly appreciating the impact that they may have on our physical, emotional and mental wellbeing. The ability to not only build and maintain good habits but also break bad ones is an essential life skill that helps to give us purpose, satisfaction and the opportunity to create meaningful change within ourselves and those around us.

Having the insight to recognise when things are not going well because of consistent behaviours, or an absence of, is just as important. We sometimes lack this insight not because our motivation is obscured but because our environment facilitates or encourages certain habits for proximal success, rather than widespread or longer-term satisfaction and impact. In modern society we often find ourselves with work at the top of our priority list. It does bring home the proverbial bacon. But how many of us can say that we maintain good habits not only at our job but also around it? And even if we can see where things are going wrong, can we change them? Do we have the desire to? Do we have the capacity, the skills and the strategies to?

At the core of our vocation as health professionals, we have dedicated ourselves to assisting and helping people. Individuals often come to us with an injury, seeking some form of intervention to improve their health, as they cannot do so on their own. And whilst our role may be inclusive of a wide range of treatment options, fundamentally we are helping that person create a positive behaviour change: to exercise for a purpose, to look after their body through various self-care strategies, to improve their self-efficacy and physical capacity so that they may return to their normal habits and participate in what is important to them.

Developing habits that help to create the life you want to live and become the person you want to be can be transformative. Everyone will value actions and behaviours differently, depending on their own circumstances and motivations. It is important not to lose sight of your own amongst the crowd. For the purpose of this book, we are going to focus on three interrelated areas where habits are often explored in the real world: recovery, sleep and nutrition.

Exercise has been thoroughly studied and its benefits are seemingly endless. Despite this, many of us find it difficult to consistently perform exercise, often foregoing it in favour of something else that makes us feel emotionally better at the time. Often, we implement recovery strategies even less so. We may contemplate engaging in activities to recover, whether it be physically or mentally, but how do we incorporate this into our routine?

Research into good sleep habits and the impact they have on our overall wellbeing has increased over these last few decades, as sleep has been shown to have a positive effect on cognitive ability and emotion regulation whilst having a strong interrelationship with exercise.

Nutrition relative to habits can be easily overlooked as it is often oversimplified into eating regularly at three main intervals across the day, interspersed with smaller meals or snacks of some description. However, nutrition's relevance and complexity when exploring habits for success is not to be underestimated, given the effects it can have on sleep quality, exercise capacity and other factors crucial for day-to-day results.

Boundaries, Burnout and Self-Discipline

Instilling daily habits into distinct aspects of your life in an almost ritualistic approach can provide you with the opportunity to be more efficient and more impactful with your footprint, both personally and professionally. Habits are a huge part of Tim Ferriss' lifestyle design method (Ferriss, 2011). We encourage you to work on the small wins and achievable habits first. Put your focus into the areas that will allow you to both reap the early rewards of your labour and have the most significant feedforward effect.

Establishing boundaries is a key action that you need to adaptively apply in your career to ensure that you do not become overwhelmed and overworked. The creation of such boundaries can assist in forming good habits effectively. Boundary setting, whether in relation to your personal life, work or otherwise, will require frequent reflection, adjustment and re-evaluation. It is okay to not get things right the first time, or the second. This adaptive learning process is helping you adjust your actions, thoughts and emotions into a habit that will be more meaningful and more successful.

When boundaries are not respected, or wilfully broken too often, you may begin to experience 'burnout'. As defined and examined in Chapter 1, burnout is an issue for striving physiotherapists who do not monitor and take action to improve their wellbeing. It is vitally important to be able to recognise the signs of burnout, not only in yourself but also in your colleagues, as these signs are often dismissed or overshadowed. The process and manifestation of burnout is very individualised, but each presentation often shares any number of characteristics, real or perceived, that are a result of the environment in which we are 'trapped'.

It is crucial that you monitor yourself for any of these signs and, if present, ask questions, reflect and analyse your practice, behaviours and emotions. Restoration of balance, habits and wellbeing practices will not only allow you to overcome any feelings of burnout in time but also help you spot and resolve burnout earlier. These concepts surrounding burnout are further explored in Chapter 1.

Another integral concept within the scope of habits is that of self-discipline. This is usually represented by a person's motivation, desire and willingness to pursue something better for themselves. Despite any factors that may function as a barrier or deterrent, their actions exemplify genuine follow-through on their intentions. Self-discipline can be the differentiating factor for those who succeed in their academic endeavours and performance (Gong et al., 2009; Duckworth & Seligman, 2005).

Developing self-discipline, like many things, takes time and focus. Starting with something small, yet both meaningful and achievable, will help provide you with the opportunity to practise your ability to remain disciplined, before increasing the challenge and diversifying your focus to other areas of your life, personal or professional. It is important to understand the intrinsic motivating factors behind developing your discipline. Are you simply completing those extra hours or duties at work because you feel perceived pressure to do so? Or are you doing it to help you to meet your career objectives or feel satisfied with the impact you have created from your day's work? When you better understand the 'why', you will find the 'how' much simpler.

Ryan Holiday's book *Discipline Is Destiny* defines three key areas he believes we need to instil discipline within – mind, body and spirit (Holiday, 2022; ideated in Fig. 3.1). And within those areas, there are important steps to improving satisfaction and sense of worth and achievement.

1. Controlling your body: Feel your body's responses to challenges and learn from that feedback.
2. Moderating your mind: Giving in to impulses or chances for instant gratification can be unrewarding and empty.
3. Actualisation: Stay calm, show up, do the work and show compassion to yourself and others.

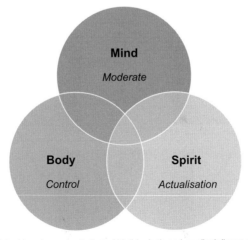

Fig. 3.1 Visual representation of Holiday's three key disciplinary areas.

When we do not appropriately identify barriers, nor have sufficient strategies to overcome them, self-discipline practices may take a backward step. This coincides with burnout in many ways. Learning and understanding that these obstacles are a part of life, a part of every career and workplace, is an important lesson. Once acknowledged and accepted, this lesson will help you to stay professional and keep your resolve, even in the toughest of circumstances. Self-discipline is not about deprivation or complete sacrifice; rather it is being in control of your actions, thoughts and emotions so that your journey has both opportunities and purpose.

Habit Formation

It is important that your habits are sustainable so that they can realistically be maintained on a regular basis. Habits should be used to improve your work-life balance and optimise your time and enjoyment – they should not just be about contributing to 'survival'. Understanding the concept of habit formation is an essential skill; without this, the application can be increasingly arduous.

Further reading into the topic of habit formation and behaviour change should be essential within your continued professional development, and we strongly recommend delving deeper into this area of study. There are several important concepts raised by eminent thought leaders in the field of habits such as James Clear, Charles Duhigg and BJ Fogg.

In his best-selling book *Atomic Habits*, world-renowned blogger and public speaker James Clear introduces a 'habit loop' concept (Fig. 3.2) (Clear, 2018). He suggests that we should make the cue obvious, make the craving attractive, make the response easy and make the reward also attractive. The opposite also applies when trying to break unattractive habits: make the cue invisible, make the craving unattractive, make the response hard and make the reward unattractive. As Clear says, 'You do not rise to the level of your goals. You fall to the level of your systems' (Clear, 2018, p. 27).

Charles Duhigg (2014), reporter for the *New York Times* and writer for the *New Yorker*, proposes a similar model (Fig. 3.3), where the cue is a visual, physical, emotional or environmental trigger that tells your brain to initiate a habit. The craving is the motivation due to the reward you will get by engaging in the habit. This is first followed by the routine, the physical and/or mental

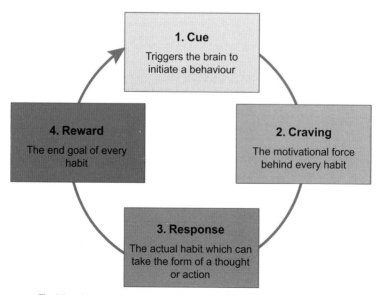

Fig. 3.2   Visual representation of Clear's 'habit loop' from *Atomic habits.*

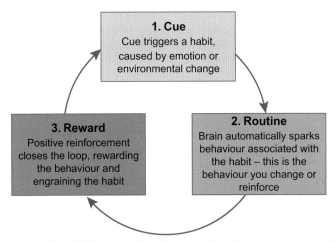

Fig. 3.3 Visual representation of Duhigg's model from *The power of habit*. (Adapted with permission from Duhigg, C. [2014]. *The power of habit: Why we do what we do in life and business*. Random House Trade Paperbacks.)

response to the cue, rounded off with the reward, with your brain being signalled to repeat the habit. Of note, Duhigg's strategy for habit formation has one key difference, and that is to try to change the routine that is within the loop, aiming to create the right individualised routines using pre-existing triggers.

B. J. Fogg (2020), the esteemed Stanford professor, explores a behaviour model in his book *Tiny Habits*. The model is conceptualised through the B=MAP principles (Fig. 3.4).

- B = behaviour, an action that somebody does
- M = motivation, sensation, anticipation, belonging – our intrinsic drive
- A = ability, how easy is it for someone to do something at that moment in time
- P = prompts, triggers and cues

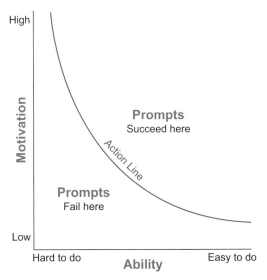

Fig. 3.4 Visual representation of Fogg's B=MAP model from *Tiny habits*. (With permission from Fogg, B. J. [2020]. *Tiny habits: The small changes that change everything*. Houghton Mifflin Harcourt.)

Fogg suggests that people tend to struggle as they look to impart substantial changes over a brief period. The concept of tiny habits combined with 'anchoring' highlights the prospect of starting with something you do once a day, with little effort, taking less than 30 seconds, using this as a building block to compound further habits. Using this automatic, low-effort behaviour as an anchor to which you can then 'stack' on further habits provides your routine with a logical, organised sequence where one habit simply leads into another.

Creating good habits and eradicating or replacing suboptimal ones are important not only for you as a healthcare professional but also for you to instil and share with those under your care. Effectively treating any individual across any range of patient populations requires elevated levels of skill around behaviour change. Understanding habit formation will empower you to enter a discussion and collaboratively create strategies to improve their own habits, aligning with their goals and desires and improving their potential outcome.

Goal Setting and Systems

Goal setting is an important conduit of habits; however, prioritising effective systems and processes that align with your purpose and values will make achieving those goals simpler and more meaningful. Overfocusing on goal setting creates a specificity and rigidity that can drive you towards failure rather than success. Goals often need to be adaptable and reframed throughout the process, and you must be accepting of both this and the fact that your goals may change across your journey. By establishing habits, systems and processes, any event, whether it is progress or a setback, is still guided by those founding principles which hold you in the right direction and will lead to more fulfilment and satisfaction.

Remember, goal achievement is only momentary and often replaced with something else just as quickly. Goals may help you set the direction in which you wish to act, but systems will allow you to make true progress. Focusing too solely on the goal itself can often impact not only the outcome but also the emotional experience as if we cannot feel happiness or satisfaction until the goal is achieved. It can be likened to treating the symptoms of a condition but not the cause. Hence, it is crucial to remember that if you work to fix the inputs, then the outputs produce the desired consequences organically. Do not underestimate the compounding effect that you can achieve through the accumulation of seemingly small improvements and adjustments to both your personal and professional life.

Motivation

Critically acclaimed writer Steven Pressfield (2012) said that at some point, the pain of not doing it became greater than the pain of doing it. Whether it is in the form of an object, action or event, the concept of reward regularly drives human action. The feeling we experience from the idea of a reward can be immensely powerful and motivates us to want to act. However, at times there may be a near-complete absence of methods that help you to get or stay motivated. That is until we break through the mental threshold that may be holding us back as we weigh the cost of our choices to act or not to act.

Motivation can be scheduled to maximise its outcome. By setting a schedule, the likelihood that you will follow through with your proposed actions is increased. Rather than wasting time or resources on the decision-making process, let the decisions be made for you ahead of time in a ritualistic manner. This simplifies the idea of starting a behaviour or habit, so you can put all of yourself, all your motivation, to complete it, even when it becomes difficult.

The Goldilocks Rule is a phenomenon that suggests peak motivation can be experienced when you are working on a challenge that is at the cusp of your ability and is key to maintaining long-term motivation. It is also imperative that your progress is measured, not only against the challenge or the task in front of you but also by the feedback you are receiving. If these components do not align, then your desire may wane and the potential boost in happiness that coincides with peak motivation may disappear.

The idea of using an appropriately challenging task or directive links to our own central reward system. Dopamine, a key neurotransmitter within our brain's circuitry, has been referred to as the 'molecule of possibilities' (Lieberman & Lon, 2018). It is released by neurons when we expect to or receive a reward and can enhance the memories and learning associated with that experience. The amount of dopamine-related signalling is directly correlated to the expected reward – if the reward is greater than anticipated, more dopamine is released, whilst the opposite occurs in the antagonistic scenario. Think of someone who has walked through your door at work, who you have been helping for weeks without a real end in sight. Then one day, unexpectedly, they inform you that they no longer have pain, they are performing activities that are meaningful to them and they have their quality of life back. That sense of satisfaction and relief, that rush, is driven by dopamine. The neuroscience behind this phenomenon has been extensively researched. To learn more about the science of 'chasing your dreams', we recommend reading *Dopamine Nation* by Dr. Anna Lembke (2023) and *The Molecule of More* (Lieberman & Lon, 2018) or, for the auditory learner, exploring the work of Andrew Huberman (2022) based at Stanford University (Huberman Lab podcast).

Motivation must be coupled with habits; otherwise there is no result, no tangible learning, just an emotion, thought or desire. Motivation may get you to the starting line, but without a bridge between motivation and habits, you may not reach the finish line.

Sleep

We must reset our physical and mental state every day to create the impact most of us desire. We are self-reliant to ensure that we give ourselves a chance for this reset to occur each night. It is thought that the human body can last without sleep for only up to 11 days, with the physical and cognitive signs of deprivation starting much quicker, usually within 72 hours. Our sleep cycle is researched and is made up of two main components:

1. NREM sleep: This can be comparable to our wake reflective periods and is where we process facts, skills and learning.
2. REM sleep: This is where we integrate past experiences with new ones. It is linked strongly to the emotional aspects of the human brain and is said to lead to increased creativity.

Individually, we all have different sleep demands, although the general recommendation in adulthood is 7 to 8 hours per night. There is variance with respect to this, as some people may only require 6 hours whilst others require 10 hours. Life in the 21st century is not particularly conducive to suitable sleep hygiene. We are surrounded by technological distractions, artificial lights and lengthy periods indoors. The role and application of habits around sleep are being investigated more frequently and in more depth, particularly around performance. But we must be mindful to not allow this research to remain solely in academic papers. Renowned sleep consultant Anna West mentions that her mission is to transform these learnings into 'implementable strategies that can help people change bad habits and ultimately make them understand how they can use sleep as a repeated performance enhancer'. The work is there, and we need to employ the lessons from it.

There are numerous methods to manipulate your pre- and post-sleep routine in order to optimise performance (Fig. 3.5), and it is suggested that you commence their application within 90 minutes of your actual bedtime. Your natural circadian rhythm must be considered when exploring habits, as these natural processes may define your body's ability or receptiveness to certain

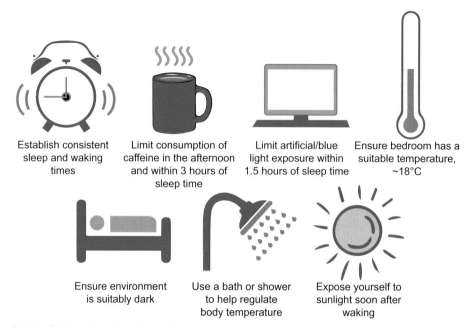

Fig. 3.5 Evidence-based practices to improve your sleep quality and quantity. (With permission from Centers for Disease Control and Prevention [CDC]. [2022, September 13]. *Tips for better sleep.* Available at https://www.cdc.gov/sleep/about_sleep/sleep_hygiene.html. Accessed 2 May 2023.)

behaviours at certain times of the day depending on your level of wakefulness versus sleepiness (Littlehales, 2016). For example, the idea of a 'night owl' or a 'morning bird' when describing an individual's preference for when they perform meaningful tasks is related to their circadian chronotype. If you have been told you are a 'night owl' and you reflect on your own habitual schedule, you will see an association with completing those key tasks late at night. This is a simple yet important way to improve your performance.

Using the idea of polyphasic sleep, where you sleep in multiples of 90-minute cycles, has also been suggested to improve focus (Littlehales, 2016). Whether you sleep in a single continuous burst or a 6-hour period combined with another 90-minute nap during the day, it is important to regulate this so that you can have an appropriate balance between activity and recovery. Think about the days you have gone to work after only having 4 hours of sleep, or you missed having that afternoon nap the day before. It is highly likely that your ability to concentrate, your communication with people under your care, and the speed and quality of your work are negatively impacted, as you continually look at the clock for your next coffee break. Now compare that to a day at work where you were able to get 7.5 to 9 hours of sleep the night before – the day flies by as you are in a flow state, and you have the energy to complete those additional nonclinical tasks that are typically a chore.

We are never going to get things perfect, but we are looking to instil better habits that will improve our ability to achieve more optimal quantities and qualities of sleep so that we can experience the benefits in the waking hours of the day. 'If you just get a little bit of a better understanding of the human relationship with light and dark, you'll start to figure it out', says sport sleep coach Nick Littlehales, who has worked with Manchester United, Liverpool, Real Madrid and British cycling teams.

Nutrition

The area of nutrition is often underutilised from all facets but is closely interrelated with the areas of sleep and recovery. Chronic malnutrition or poor habits are often reflections of not coping with the stressors around you, making the body more susceptible to burnout, injuries and other negative connotations.

As health professionals, we know that nutrition is a useful topic that can be discussed at even a basic level with individuals in your network to help them build habits that create better outcomes through improved wellbeing standards. Exploring this in detail goes beyond the scope of this chapter, but we encourage you to investigate your areas of interest so that you can begin to apply them yourself and assist others.

Nutritional guidelines are often heavily promoted but should be thought of as more of a framework, given that all individuals have quite varying nutritional requirements. Habit formation principles are much the same for nutrition as they are for sleep, recovery and other daily occurrences we have discussed in this chapter. Apply your own chosen methodology to create the behaviour change and the outcomes you desire. The work of Daniel Davey, sports nutritionist for Leinster Rugby and Dublin GAA and author of best-selling books *Eat Up: Raise Your Game* and *Eat Up: The Next Level*, advocates for creating a lifestyle of effectiveness in which all controllable factors are working to improve performance, such as sleep, food and recovery. The perfect meal every now and then will not do much to make a dent in a bad lifestyle, but consistent good habits in each of these will yield exponential results that will compound over time.

As we have previously stated, we are looking for better, rather than perfect. The population you are working with, the performance requirements or the goals you have set will dictate how greatly you must chase perfection. Utilising software or applications to support your behaviours is something that can help keep you on track and consistent. David Dunne, behavioural change scientist, pro golf nutritionist and founder of the revolutionary app 'Hexis', focuses on carbohydrates as a primary fuel source and creating awareness around our individual requirements. David's goal is to help everyone realise their full potential by tailoring artificial intelligence–powered nutrition to the specific demands of your everyday life. We will all have our own needs and requirements for energy, so employing external supports such as software can greatly improve our ability to stick to routine, meal plans or positive nutritional habits. Check out his model around carb coding as an example. Undoubtedly, self-discipline combined with habit formation can be used effectively to ensure good planning is actioned, to reduce the desire or requirement for food that is merely 'convenient'.

Here are some suggestions that you may apply within your own circumstances:

1. Eat more wholesome food that is as close as possible to its natural source, reducing consumption of processed foods.
2. Try to eat the number of fruits and vegetables as suggested by standard nutritional guidelines, as well as 'eating the rainbow' to increase the range of vitamins and minerals being consumed.
3. Be aware that guidelines often underestimate the amount of protein required daily. Proteins, the building blocks of tissue regeneration, are heavily linked to recovery status. In the general population, your foundational protein consumption levels should be around 1.2 to 1.6 g/kg of your body weight daily, and up to 2 g/kg in athletic populations.
4. Ensure adequate hydration from various sources, using urination frequency and colour as a guide. Over 50% of the human body constitutes water. Requirements are again individual and environment dependent and can be affected by a number of factors – exercise/physical activity levels, diet, vitamin levels and temperature/climate exposure.
5. Consider the use of supplementation where your goals/targets require it, not simply as a replacement for consuming natural food sources.
6. Ensure an appropriate ratio of macronutrients are being consumed, with a standard breakdown often recommending 40% protein, 40% carbohydrates and 20% fats. This can then be modified depending on what you are attempting to achieve.

We must recognise the nutritional benefit that comes with eating a varied food matrix. This will allow our body systems to work more efficiently and increase the opportunities to optimise our nutritional status. Of course, we recommend food-based sources first, but sometimes supplementation can be used as an adjunct method to ensure we are obtaining what we need.

We each require a certain number of calories for basic survival. This is very individualised, as are the potential needs of any additional calories to perform and sustain activity levels above that of general functioning. A simplification of needs would state that an individual who is highly active, and/or has a higher percentage of lean muscle mass, will have a higher caloric requirement. Understanding basic principles around our basal metabolic rate (BMR) is important to ensure nutritional practices are adaptive and specific, depending on what we are aiming to achieve. For example, if you are looking to lose weight, then your calorie intake should be lower than your BMR, and vice versa if you are attempting to gain weight. There are numerous ways that you can calculate BMR, including the Harris-Benedict formula (Frankenfield *et al.*, 1998).

Males: body weight in kg × 24

Females: body weight in kg × 22

Multiply your resultant number by the appropriate factor in relation to your activity level (add in definitions for each classification). It is worth noting that people often overestimate their activity levels.

- Sedentary = 1.2
- Lightly active = 1.375
- Moderately active = 1.55
- Very active = 1.725
- Extra active = 1.9

It would be impossible to review and consolidate the entire nutritional landscape into a mere subsection of a chapter. Hopefully, the above information has sparked your interest to delve deeper into the relationship that nutrition has with habits.

Recovery

The idea of engaging in recovery practices can be uninspiring and tedious. However, the impacts can be profound and rewarding on a multitude of levels. The importance of recovery has gained significant traction, both in the literature and in application, particularly as nonphysical modalities are explored to determine their contribution to peak physical, cognitive and emotional performance. The idea of recovery can be complex as intrinsic, extrinsic, activity and environmental stressors must be balanced to allow lofty standards to be maintained.

From a physical perspective, athletes, coaches, health professionals and the like are continually seeking any advantage possible to ensure the greatest chance of success is within their grasp. These modalities may be active or passive in nature and are often the most thought of processes or techniques that contribute to recovery. A concise summary of these techniques and common applications has been detailed by the Human Kinetics group (see Fig. 3.6; Human Kinetics, 2021).

Best practice methodologies are often debated when it comes to recovery techniques, so much so that some even question whether they have any impact at all on an individual's recovery. It is important to remember that even if the application of one of the strategies does not result in a true physical or physiological change, the psychological and emotional benefit that may be achieved can have an immeasurable impact. As individuals work through recovery strategies, they will learn to understand their body more, what it needs to be nurtured and what it needs to perform. Sometimes it can be a challenge to find not only what makes you feel good but also an activity that you engage and connect with. Recovery does not have to be a chore; it can be enjoyable, reflective and meaningful conjunctively. It may take time to find what works for you, but when you do, you will have a greater appreciation for that activity and will become more likely to make it a habit because of how you feel when you engage with that process.

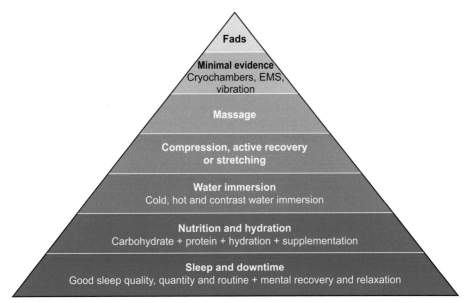

Fig. 3.6 Visual representation of a typical hierarchy of physical recovery. *EMS*, electric muscle stimulation. (With permission from French, D., Ronda, L. T. [2021]. *NSCA's essentials of sport science*, National Strength & Conditioning Association, Human Kinetics.)

Recovery may also be an opportunity to further develop strengths whilst working to improve weaknesses. For example, you may be in peak physical condition and consistently performing well within your chosen sport or profession, but psychologically and emotionally, you may be experiencing burnout or compassion fatigue. Acknowledging and being self-aware that you are experiencing any of these phenomena is a key step that will allow you to facilitate meaningful change. But that does not mean you have to take away from areas that are going well or stop focusing on your strengths. Instead, you may use those activities, which are already ingrained, important habits, as an opportunity to integrate other practices such as mindfulness, meditation or journal writing to effectively 'habit stack' and create a multimodal recovery practice for yourself.

Through the creation of habitual recovery practices, you learn how to ensure that you are ready to deal with anything that the day ahead of you may present. By focusing on your whole self and concentrating on the moment, you are likely to become aware of any potential problems before they become problems.

Reflections From Matt Bruno

When I was asked to contribute to this incredible project, I was very humbled and excited. When I was informed that I would be writing the chapter on habits, of course I said yes. But really I was asking myself, 'Why me?' My day-to-day life is chaotic as I attempt to juggle family, pets, sport, work, side projects and renovating a house – the list of things that I am trying to achieve each day just grows. Just as it does for everyone. No two days or weeks are ever the same. How can I write about my habits, which are supposed to be consistent, where there is no consistency?

It was not until I began to explore the science of habits that I reflected on my own. The things that I do each day, the thoughts that I have, the character and attitude I display, they are all habitual in their own way and have allowed me to achieve what I have. I have created my own framework and processes, whether I have realised it or not, that fundamentally allowed order to shine through what looks like disorder.

When my list gets too large, I will be the first to admit that I sacrifice sleep. It simply gives me more time to get things done. But through experience, having used this strategy since I was in high school, I now recognise the impact that it has not only on the person that I am, or could be, but also on the resulting habits and patterns. I would exercise regularly but often found myself making poor dietary choices. I had accepted that a near-constant state of physical and mental fatigue was my new normal when it really did not have to be. Eventually, I would make excuses not to exercise, prioritising anything else as I became stuck in a cycle of trying to set myself up for success and satisfaction now, instead of laying groundwork composed of consistency and value, which would set me up for longer-term benefits and more meaningful growth.

I decided that I had to change, not only to get the best out of myself but also for those around me. To make sure that I was present in the moment. Accepting that this habitual cycle I had created was not out of necessity, but because I had just accepted things as they were, was hard to admit and something I still struggle with occasionally when times get tough. However, the satisfaction that comes from not only challenging yourself to create consistency but the results and wonders you can achieve can be truly life changing. Whilst each day or week may be inconsistent, or even random, what that time is composed of is the opposite. It is deliberate, it is valuable and it is habitual.

We all value the triad of sleep, nutrition and recovery in diverse ways at contrasting times. One or all may be influenced by circumstantial factors that phase in and out with time; they may be influenced by intrinsic or extrinsic motivators, or they may be a reflection of a particular goal we are trying to achieve at any given moment. Whatever it may be, it is crucial to recognise the influence that they have on each other, the changes in behaviour they create and what the resultant habits look like. Are these the habits that best reflect you? Do they give you the chance to be the person you want to be?

Reflections From Paul Stevens

Reflecting on the start of my physiotherapy journey, regarding studying, I very much focused on quantity. I felt that the more hours I put in, the better results I would get out. Admittedly this had the desired effect, and I did achieve good grades and went on to graduate as a physiotherapist. However, looking back, the use of my time was not always efficient. I now understand the importance of focused work, ensuring the working environment is appropriate and trying to achieve a flow state when working on something that requires my full attention. In a world of distractions this is becoming more challenging to achieve. Whatever stage of your career you are in, I would strongly encourage you to read about the topic of achieving 'flow' within your work. We must focus on single tasks and direct all our attention to that task rather than trying to juggle multiple tasks. To initiate this process, it is worth doing a self-analysis of when you do your best work – for instance, are you an early bird or a night owl? If a piece of work requires creativity and important levels of focus, schedule the completion of this task when you feel that you are at your most optimal. If a task is more menial, then the scheduling is less important.

In my opinion, boundaries and work-life balance are extremely high on the priority list when we are looking at essential skills for physiotherapists, and any other profession. Reflecting upon my 14-year physiotherapist career so far, I have not always practised what I now preach. I started my career in private practice. Initially I had set start and finish times, with adequate lunch breaks and scheduled administration time. However, in the first few years of my career I did not have a good appreciation of the importance of boundaries to strike an effective work-life balance. I progressively started to extend my working day, with earlier start times and later finish times. My breaks then became shorter, or worse still, I often ate whilst travelling between clinics. I found myself getting into the habit of completing administrative tasks either early in the morning, before clinics or late at night, after clinics. I was seeing a high volume of patients, keeping the contract stakeholders happy and achieving excellent patient results, as confirmed by the audit, but I was driving myself down the road to burnout. I progressively increased my daily clinical hours from 6–8 hours up to 10–12 hours, often with an additional couple of hours of administrative tasks. I was constantly working 12- to 14-hour days. My working week followed the same progression – creeping up from 5 days, to the occasional 6 days, to the frequent 6 days and then often working 7 days a week. I can assure you that this above model is not sustainable, and from my experience it is amazingly easy to fall into the trap.

If you find yourself working 12- to 14-hour days, 5 to 7 days a week, you will quickly discover that the space for the life part of work-life balance is diminished. If you are a career-driven and achievement-focused individual, then you will inevitably, at times, find yourself overworking and pushing the work-life pendulum too far towards the work side. If this is short-lived and then you re-address the work-life balance, that can be a sustainable model. However, if this becomes a chronic state of your career, then it is not sustainable. Having an awareness of how easy it is to slip into overworking and heading towards burnout is important at any point of your career, but especially so at the start.

In 2016 I switched from working within a private practice model of work (dealing with a combination of subcontracted national health work, insurance work and athletes) to contracting work with the military. The military work had predetermined working hours and clinics with scheduled micro and macro breaks. I was suddenly back to working 8-hour clinical days, with time for administrative tasks and working 4 half-days per week. I had the opportunity for sleep, physical activity and socialising with family and friends. My energy levels, sense of fulfilment and happiness increased very quickly. I had been aware that I had been working hard, and potentially overworking, but I was unaware of just how chronically tired I had become until I realised how much better I felt with shorter working days, more sleep, more focused physical activity and more time for socialising.

It is important to remember that striking the optimal work-life balance is a continuous process that requires regular reflection, analysis and amendment. You will not always get it right, and not the first time. Find reflective practices and strategies that work for you to ensure you achieve the optimal balance.

Habits are purposefully chosen actions that you, as an individual, choose to add to your day because they are meaningful and create an impact within yourself and your larger circle. They are the invisible architecture that comprises our lives. It is important to celebrate when both your endeavour and these processes culminate into success and to reflect, learn and adapt when they do not. Habits are not designed to make things perfect but to encourage you to be present, to improve yourself, to improve your impact and to give you every chance at success and satisfaction.

Five Key Takeaways

1. Start small – look to change habits in small ways; do not underestimate the compounding effect of incremental changes.
2. Explore your environment on a deeper level. Optimise it to make desirable habits autonomous whilst reducing resistance from potential barriers.
3. Create a system of habit tracking that creates a chain reaction and satisfying process, playing on the neuroscience that helps engrain habits and makes them less effortful.
4. When looking to create, change or remove habits, it is important to consider routines, processes and the idea of behaviour change from the perspective of everyday life.
5. Show up and be consistent. We are looking to perform better slowly, not be perfect immediately. Don't underestimate the power of simply getting started.

Five Self-Directed Reflections

1. What, or who, motivates you to create change?
2. Reflecting on your end goal, what processes can you implement now to help achieve it?
3. What physical, visual or environmental cues can you utilise to optimise your behaviour?
4. Who is in your corner to keep you grounded and accountable?
5. What are the one to two actions that you can take today that will make the most impact on your path to becoming your ideal self?

References

Clear, J. (2018). *Atomic habits*. Penguin USA.

Duckworth, A. L., & Seligman, M. E. P. (2005). Self-discipline outdoes IQ in predicting academic performance of adolescents. *Psychological Science, 16*(12), 939–944. https://doi.org/10.1111/j.1467-9280.2005.01641.x.

Duhigg, C. (2014). *The power of habit: Why we do what we do in life and business*. Random House Trade Paperbacks.

Ferriss, T. (2011). *The 4-hour work week*. Crown Publishing Group.

Fogg, B. J. (2020). *Tiny habits: The small changes that change everything*. Houghton Mifflin Harcourt.

Frankenfield, D. C., Muth, E. R., & Rowe, W. A. (1998). The Harris-Benedict studies of human basal metabolism. *Journal of the American Dietetic Association, 98*(4), 439–445. https://doi.org/10.1016/s0002-8223(98)00100-x.

French, D., & Ronda, L. T. (2021). *NSCA's essentials of sport science*. National Strength & Conditioning Association, Human Kinetics.

Gong, Y., Rai, D., Beck, J. E., & Heffernan, N. T. (2009). *Does self-discipline impact students' knowledge and learning?* In *Proceedings of the 2nd International Conference on Educational Data Mining*. Cordoba, Spain.

Hawk, R. (2022). *The pursuit of excellence: The uncommon behaviors of the world's most productive achievers*. McGraw Hill.

Holiday, R. (2022). *Discipline is destiny: The power of self-control*. Portfolio/Penguin, an imprint of Penguin Random House LLC.

Huberman, A. (2022). Science based tools for increasing happiness (No. 98) [Audio podcast episode]. In *The Huberman Lab*. Scicomm Media. Available at https://www.youtube.com/watch?v=LTGGyQS1fZE. Accessed 7 March 2024.

Human Kinetics. (2021). *What are the best recovery strategies for athletes?* Available at https://humankinetics.me/2021/07/15/what-are-the-best-recovery-strategies-for-athletes/. Accessed 20 January 2024.

Lembke, A. (2023). *Dopamine nation: Finding balance in the age of indulgence*. Dutton, an imprint of Penguin Random House LLC.

Lieberman, D. Z., & Long, M. E. (2018). *The molecule of more: How a single chemical in your brain drives love sex and creativity—and will determine the fate of the human race*. BenBella Books.

Littlehales, N. (2016). *Sleep: Change the way you sleep with this 90-minute read*. Penguin Life.

Pressfield, S. (2012). *The war of art: Break through the blocks and win your inner creative battles*. Black Irish Entertainment, LLC.

Further Reading

Headspace. (n.d.). How to sleep better. Available at https://www.headspace.com/sleep/how-to-sleep-better. Accessed 2 January 2024.

Science for Sports (2024). *Recovery archives*. Available at https://www.scienceforsport.com/category/recovery/. Accessed 2 March 2024.

World Health Organization. (2022). *International classification of diseases (ICD) revision 11*.

Relationships

CHAPTER 4

Better Communication – Intentional Listening, Empathy and Feedback

Nicol van Dyk ■ Phil Glasgow

'No matter how smart, talented, driven, or passionate you are, your success depends on your ability to effectively negotiate …. Negotiation isn't just a business tool – it's a life skill.'
– Christopher Voss, *New York Times* best-selling author of *Never Split the Difference* and former FBI hostage negotiator

Introduction

What is it like to be listened to? Can you think of a time when you have felt that the other person 'got it'? They understand you, the issue and what you are trying to achieve.

At its core, our therapeutic interaction is about shaping and shifting how individuals and groups attend to and subsequently respond to a situation or condition. Many therapists are unable to recognise, let alone change, the structural habits of paying attention. Learning to recognise the habits of attention in any culture requires, among other things, a particular kind of listening.

Listening can be narrowly defined as an auditory process of gathering information from sound. But we have come to experience listening as the active process of receiving and responding to spoken (and unspoken) messages, experiences and emotions. As the poet Alice Duer Miller writes, 'Listening means taking a vigorous, human interest in what is being told us. You can listen like a blank wall or like a splendid auditorium where every sound comes back fuller and richer' (Nordquist, 2020).

Communicating well matters, as it remains crucial for successful therapeutic encounters (Gask & Usherwood, 2002) and may impact your interactions and outcomes. A proficient subjective assessment is fundamental to creating a good interpersonal relationship, as well as information exchange and optimal professional decision-making (Chester *et al.*, 2014; Ong *et al.*, 1995; Stewart & Stasser, 1995).

The early stages of the therapeutic encounter are also when patients present their problems to the therapist. This first opportunity is important for a successful outcome and often is the only time in a medical encounter that patients are given the opportunity to describe their condition in their own words and address their personal agenda (Heritage & Robinson, 2006). But when patients are invited into the therapeutic relationship as a co-designer of their own outcomes, and given the opportunity to participate, they are more likely to work alongside the therapist and, better yet, have increased satisfaction with the outcome (Glueckauf, 1993; Payton *et al.*, 1998) Poor communication may have the opposite effect, specifically nonadherence or poor compliance with a chosen treatment (Zolnierek & DiMatteo, 2009). Therefore, the clinician's communication skills are vital in establishing a good interpersonal relationship with patients, creating a welcoming environment and enabling patients to freely express their issues (Chester *et al.*, 2014).

In our everyday interactions with our patients in the clinic, we are often already planning our treatment option(s) within the first few minutes of a session (more than enough time to do a thorough subjective assessment). We know the pathology (all of them behave predictably, of course), we know the treatments (now at expert level after that weekend workshop), we run a quick algorithm in our mind (free of any heuristics, naturally), check against our clinical experience (whatever it is at that stage seems plenty) and decide on the best 'evidence-based' course of action. Sound familiar? This is the trap we all sometimes fall into and can avoid if we understand the value of building a relationship with the patient to allow effective communication (van Dyk *et al.*, 2019). We will explore listening as one of the key components of creating a working alliance with your patient, and how you might assess and develop the crucial skill of listening.

We first share some of our personal experiences to help set the scene for this chapter, and we encourage you to think about how you want your patients to feel when they leave a consultation with you.

Reflections From Nicol van Dyk

When I was 23 years old, I had a serious spinal injury. After an unfortunate collision in a rugby match, I was upended and landed badly on my neck. The immediate care was excellent, and I was rushed to hospital. Several investigations later would confirm I had broken my neck – a hairline fracture of C5, with complete rupture of the anterior longitudinal, posterior longitudinal and spinal ligaments, as well as a ruptured intervertebral disc. It was serious, but fortunately with no spinal cord involvement.

A double fusion was performed, and I was immobilised in a collar for 3 months, with lots of rehab to come. You'd think that as a then-third-year physiotherapy student I was going to benefit from understanding the pathoanatomical process, the surgery and the likely rehabilitation journey to come. But I was overcome with anxiety, uncertainty and fear for what this might mean for the rest of my life. Effectively my rugby career was over (that didn't bother me, although I loved the game and didn't participate in any other sports or activities at the time), but would I still be able to be a good physio? Would it affect my daily life? Would I have pain, and would it get worse later on? These thoughts occupied my mind as I went for my first follow-up consultation with the surgeon. And so, I asked him the obvious question: 'Will I be able to go bungee jumping?'

He was furious at me. Why would I want to do that? Did I not realise the (unnecessary) risks this would represent, and he declared that it would be very likely I'd need surgery again before I'm 30 years old. He didn't get it. What I was really trying to ask him (by thinking of the riskiest thing

I've ever done) is, 'Will I be okay?' He wasn't listening. He wasn't paying attention to any of the subtle (or not-so-subtle) cues I was providing. This experience has stuck with me and shaped my own understanding of how important it is to create trust and communicate well in any circumstance, but especially in our therapeutic interaction.

Reflections From Phil Glasgow

Following a significant cycling crash a few years ago that left me with a fractured acetabulum and pelvis and a nasty head injury, I had a series of consultations with various healthcare providers. The experiences were mixed (to say the least). At times I felt frustrated that the practitioner hadn't really gotten what I was trying to ask and that I was just another in a busy clinic. I also recall a particular consultation with a very experienced consultant physician. She had been working for many years and was a formidable presence in the medical department, yet she had the ability to make me feel like I was the sole focus of her attention for the duration of our consultation.

It felt like she really wanted to understand me, my context and the challenges I was facing. She was intent on working with me to find a solution. I clearly remember the power of her simple question: What is your greatest concern in all of this? This question cut through my bravado to the main point; it was the starting point for discussions on my future in sport and my future career. While I didn't leave with all the answers, I did leave with the confidence that we were doing everything we could.

The Working Alliance – Fostering Presence and Connection in the Clinical Encounter

Time constraints, technology and administrative demands of modern medicine often impede the human connection that is central to clinical care and contribute to physician and patient dissatisfaction. Zulman *et al.* (2020) identified five practices that promote clinician presence, a state of awareness, focus and attention with the intent to understand patients. And this lies at the heart of fostering presence and connection with patients in the clinical encounter.

1. Prepare with intention: Are you prepared for a meaningful interaction?
   Familiarise yourself with the patient you are about to meet. Create a ritual to focus your attention before a visit.
2. Listen intently and completely: What does your patient say when uninterrupted?
   Sit down, lean forward and position yourself to listen. Don't interrupt. Your patient is your most valuable source of information.
3. Agree on what matters most: What are your patient's health goals, now and in the future?
   Find out what your patient cares about and incorporate these priorities into the visit agenda.
4. Connect with the patient's story: How can you contribute positively to your patient's journey?
   Consider the circumstances that influence your patient's health. Acknowledge your patient's efforts and celebrate successes.
5. Explore emotional cues: What can you learn from the patient's emotions?
   Tune in. Notice, name and validate your patient's emotions to become a trusted partner.

Consistent themes appear in the literature regarding effective therapeutic relationships. Common characteristics such as trust (Alvey & Barclay, 2007; Baron & Morin, 2009; Jowett *et al.*, 2012; O'Broin & Palmer, 2006), openness (Boyce *et al.*, 2010; Lai & McDowell, 2016; Sun *et al.*, 2013) and empathy (Rogers, 2016) are highlighted as important factors and form the basis of various descriptions of these types of relationships. These factors and their importance are perhaps best captured in the idea of 'the working alliance'.

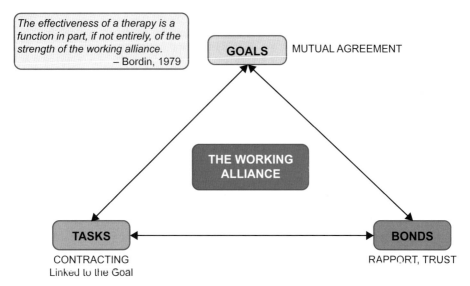

Fig. 4.1   The working alliance.

The Working Alliance

Bordin (1979, p. 254) first described the working alliance as 'the collaboration between the client and therapist built upon the development of an attachment bond alongside a mutual commitment to the goals and task'. At its heart, the working alliance is seen as a collaboration, an alliance of equals who work together to achieve an agreed outcome. Baron and Morin (2009) suggest that the emphasis on collaboration distinguishes the working alliance from other therapeutic models as it highlights the interdependence of the therapist and the client in the development of the alliance. The authors propose that the working alliance is the most robust predictive factor for therapeutic success.

Based on the three main components of *goals, tasks and bond* (Fig. 4.1), Horvath and Greenberg (1989) developed the working alliance inventory (WAI) to measure the strength of the working alliance. The WAI assesses the level of agreement regarding tasks and goals and the quality of the bond (in terms of the empathy, attractiveness, expertness and trustworthiness of the therapist) and has been used by many as a proxy for relationship quality (e.g., De Haan, 2012).

The term 'working alliance' is often referred to in healthcare as the 'therapeutic alliance'. Several studies have shown the positive effect of the therapeutic alliance on outcomes across a range of medical settings including physiotherapy (Martin, *et al.,* 2000), ulcer disease (Kaplan *et al.,* 1989) and diabetes (Lee & Lin, 2009). It has also been shown to have a strong positive correlation with outcomes related to pain, disability, physical health, mental health and patient satisfaction (Ferreira *et al.,* 2013; Fuentes *et al.,* 2014; Hall *et al.,* 2010).

Relationship as a Mediating Factor

The therapeutic relationship can be seen as the starting point for all interventions (Wampold, 2015). In a review outlining the contextual common factor model, the bond between client and therapist was identified as the foundation for the effective function of the common factors of collaboration, empathy, alliance, positive regard and empathy (Wampold, 2015). When we consider

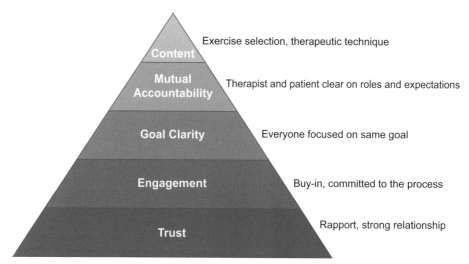

Fig. 4.2 Common factors that determine successful therapeutic interactions. (Based on principles outlined in Lewin, K. (1951). *Field theory in social science: Selected theoretical papers* [edited by Dorwin Cartwright]. Harpers.)

the literature related to coaching (Elkin, 2007; Rogers, 2016), we may draw some inferences in the therapeutic encounter from the following common factors (Fig. 4.2) in a therapeutic relationship (in descending order of importance).

1. Trust: the ability of the practitioner to create a climate of warmth, acceptance and rapport
2. Engagement: the nature of the 'therapeutic alliance'
3. Goal clarity: the context in which the client seeks help and whether they have supportive people in their lives
4. Mutual accountability: client and practitioner believing equally in the plausibility of any approaches that are used
5. Content: the kinds of techniques used

The therapist-patient relationship, as understood by the working alliance, can play a mediating role in achieving improved patient self-efficacy (Baron & Morin, 2009). The mediating influence of relationship upon therapist-patient matching (commonality, compatibility, credibility) and treatment outcomes (satisfaction/utility, treatment programme) is clear (Boyce *et al.*, 2010). This mediating role of relationship is significant and resonates with the concept of 'relationship as field' described by Pelham (2015, p. 176). He quotes Lewin (1951), who states:

> '*Whether or not a certain type of behaviour occurs depends not on the presence or absence of one fact or a number of facts viewed in isolation, but upon the constellation of the specific field as a whole.* The "meaning" of the single fact depends upon its position in the field.' *(Emphasis added)*

The idea that any specific behaviour is given meaning by virtue of its position in the field is important. If the relationship is, as Pelham suggests, a field co-created by the therapist and patient, then meaning is found in reference to the relationship. Achievement of goals and tasks emerges (or becomes figural) from the therapeutic relationship.

In a study using the coaching behaviour questionnaire, De Haan *et al.* (2012) asked coaches to identify what qualities they really appreciate in a coach. The top three qualities reported were listening, understanding and encouragement – all aspects related to relationship. And this rings true for the therapist as well. Further evidence of the importance of relationship was presented by Gyllensten and Palmer (2007), who identified trust, a sound working relationship and a sense of sharing between coach and client as key determinants of outcome.

Trust

Trust is frequently identified as the foundation for effective relationships, described as the most fundamental element required to create a safe space and facilitate openness (Pelham, 2015, p. 176). Trust enables patients to feel safe and confident enough to disclose information about their needs and weaknesses (Jowett *et al.*, 2012). Boyce *et al.* (2010) state that 'the relationship between the client and therapist is one of the most essential processes of therapy' and have identified four key processes in establishing relationship: trust, rapport, commitment and collaboration.

Relationship plays a central role in therapeutic outcomes and is a key mediator of other benefits. Therapy has a significant positive effect on patient behavioural change, and that therapist-patient relationship (or working alliance) correlates with the attainment of these goals.

Understanding the Effects of Relationship – Moving From Simplicity to Complexity

Many studies adopt a reductionist approach that seeks to identify a linear causal relationship between therapeutic outcomes and specific inputs. In simple linear systems, the observed final system's global behaviour is directly related to the sum of the contribution of its individual parts (the law of superposition). But is the therapeutic interaction a simple linear relationship where the outputs are merely the sum of the various inputs? Or is therapy better described as a complex and dynamic interaction between therapist and patient where, as Gestalt theory would suggest, the whole is more than (or something different from) the sum of the individual parts?

Existing models of therapy tend to link inputs to outcomes without discriminating the theoretical distance between the two, or even considering the role of other mediating/moderating components in the relationship (adapted from Sonesh *et al.*, 2015). The idea that inputs may have a different distance from outcomes is important. If the concept of distance is accepted, it is not possible to accurately define causal mediating relationships in what appears to be a multivariate, interdependent system.

Complexity theory may be helpful in enhancing our understanding of the role of relationships. In a complex system, elements are so connected that they produce outcomes that would not be achievable by the elements alone. Similarly, if the system were reduced to its parts, it would no longer exist. The therapeutic relationship represents dynamic complexity where cause and effect are subtle and develop over time. Given that it is impossible to effectively map every aspect of a complex relationship, therapeutic outcomes may be understood as emergent patterns that can be difficult to predict and not proportional to specific inputs (von Bertalanffy, 1969). Both complexity theory and Gestalt recognise that the actual relationship is distinct from its parts and is dependent upon the context of the system (or relationship).

Repeated interaction between therapist and patient creates patterns that cause the nature of the interaction to change and adapt. For example, as the relationship evolves, the nature of the interaction changes, which in turn changes how the relationship is perceived and produces different outcomes. Learning to pay attention to the patient and the quality of the relationship will help therapists become more skilled at co-creating positive outcomes with their patients.

Listening is far more than the capture of auditory input and goes much deeper than merely hearing what someone has to say. As Heraclitus points out, 'Most people sleep-walk through life, not understanding what is going on about them. Yet experience of words and deeds can enlighten those who are receptive to their meaning'. Listening is about being receptive to the meaning of the words and deeds that can enlighten. In order to help us navigate this complexity without giving into reductionist fallacy, we must always be attending to our patients and developing our listening skills in ways that will strengthen the therapeutic alliance we are building with our patients.

What Does Listening Look Like in the Clinical Environment?

Alarmingly, physicians only listen to a patient's concerns for a median of 11 seconds (Singh Ospina *et al.*, 2019). Physiotherapists are no better, interrupting patients between 19.9 and 45.2 seconds depending on the type of question asked (Chester *et al.*, 2014). It demonstrates how we are rarely able to set the scene, open up and let someone share their story with us. Adding to this, persons seeking our consultation are equipped with self-obtained knowledge about their condition or diagnosis. This might include a mix of honest, appropriately searched and researched information, as well as a collection of anecdotes and opinions. By carefully listening, clinicians can identify these different lanes of information and create a foundation of trust with the person (O'Keeffe *et al.*, 2016).

To achieve true integration and connectedness, behavioural learning is key. As van Dyk *et al.* (2019) writes, 'That which you discover you will more deeply own than that which I declare'. Too often, confident declarations are made in our assessment and treatment instead of asking probing and open questions. We must take on a role of facilitating the co-discovery of the person's best outcome. Facilitating the journey of discovery will not only provide greater insight into what is needed from you as a therapist but also help to further deepen the relationship with the person. If the subjective assessment is performed well, the true benefit can lie in minimal guidance of behaviour, training, exercise or adaptations in daily activities.

Different Ways of Listening and Why You Need Them All

Patients experience improved outcomes if they feel they are 'taken seriously', which often reflects the practitioner being attentive and interested in what they are saying (van Dyk *et al.*, 2019). Otto Scharmer provides clear insights on four different types of listening: downloading, factual, empathic and generative listening (Scharmer, 2008).

If you identify with downloading, what you hear confirms what you already know, seeking to reconfirm habitual judgements. When listening factually, the focus is on what is novel or disconfirming in what you hear. You allow the data to talk to you and are attentive to the responses you get. If the listener becomes empathetic, there is a shift from the clinicians to the experience horizon of the patient. This type of listening attempts to better understand the perspective of the person we listen to and creates resonance that builds trust. Ultimately, when generative listening occurs, both the clinician and patient can be themselves and share truthfully and transparently. Preconceived ideas are let go, and the interaction becomes open to a new field of possibilities.

Different Types of Listening (Scharmer, 2008; van Dyk *et al.*, 2019)

- Downloading: 'Yeah, I know that already'
  This type of listening is when what you hear confirms what you already know, and you are seeking only to reconfirm habitual judgements.
- Factual: 'Ooh, look at that'
  This is when you are able to switch off your inner voice of judgement and focus on what is novel or disconfirming in what you hear. As Scharmer says, 'You let the data talk to you', and we might call this a scientific way of listening. Asking questions and being attentive to the responses you get are key features.
- Empathic: 'Let me reflect on what I hear you saying and feeling'
  This represents a deeper level of listening, characterised by a shift from the clinician's horizon of thought and assessment to the experience horizon of the patient. This type of listening

attempts to better understand the perspective of the person we listen to; we are literally em-pathos, entering into their suffering their perspective. Reflective listening at this level creates resonance that builds trust.

■ Generative: 'I am connected to something larger than myself, and open to the unknown emergence of the interaction'
This posture is fuelled by open curiosity and a sense that the listening interaction can have something unique emerge. A deeper connection is formed in both directions and the person feels that they can be themselves, sharing truthfully and transparently. Both parties let go of preconceived ideas and become open to a new field of possibilities. With this approach we increase the possibility to identify with the patient's needs and how to best respond – an emerging understanding between you and the person. It is a creative process that allows you to adapt to each individual's unique context and needs within the therapeutic alliance.

An important starting point is to remember that people have the capability to take responsibil-ity for, and make decisions about, their own lives, rather than someone else doing this for them. The goal therefore is to build self-awareness and responsibility based on the belief that an indi-vidual's willingness to embrace change increases when there is greater awareness of the assump-tions, belief systems and behaviours that govern action.

What Does Good (Listening) Sound Like?

When we think of listening in the therapeutic alliance, we are not only thinking about what we hear but also being present to the person and listening with our whole selves – attending to ener-getic signals from the person and listening with your head, your heart and your gut, giving all your senses a chance to contribute to what you are hearing and how to listen.

A generative listener is an active listener – withholding judgement while paying attention to what is being said and, more often, what is not being said. Curious about and open to the person's views, you want to understand the point of view being provided. Ask questions to clarify what's being said, use words and phrases that are neutral, be truly interested and open to the response and changing your own mind. Here are four narrative descriptions of good listening (Zenger & Folkman, 2016).

Good Listening Is Much More Than Being Silent While the Other Person Talks

The best listeners develop the discernment of knowing how to periodically ask questions that promote discovery and insight. These questions gently challenge old assumptions but do so in a constructive way. Actively listening is not sitting in silence while nodding along, but rather consistently viewing it as a two-way dialogue, rather than a 'speaker-with-an-audience-of-one' monologue. Asking questions (often just one) tells the speaker the listener has not only heard what was said but comprehended it well enough to want additional information.

Good Listening Includes Exchanges That Contribute to the Person's Sense of Self

In active, generative listening, the conversation is experienced as positive, even if it deals with pain or despair. Good listeners make the other person feel supported, convey confidence in them and set a safe environment, allowing a person to share their story completely and discuss issues and differences openly.

Good Listening Is a Collaboration

There is no predetermined destination, and neither party is drawn into being 'correct' or assuming authority. An authentic and reciprocal approach allows feedback from the listener and the person sharing and a mutual understanding aimed at discovering insights that may lead to better outcomes, rather than winning an argument.

Good Listeners Know How to Nudge

Understanding when and how to make suggestions is the key component here. And this is not a starting point. In fact, your first encounter may lead to no suggestions whatsoever or subtle ones, like drawing the shades to allow a more soothing environment or encouraging someone to use their own words. It is imperative to meet the person where they are and steer the conversation so that you are able to get the information you need, but also the lived experience of the person becomes clear. As Zenger and Folkman state, 'Someone who is silent for the whole conversation and then jumps in with a suggestion may not be seen as credible. Someone who seems combative or critical and then tries to give advice may not be seen as trustworthy'.

Listening invariably includes some feedback provided in a way others would accept and that opens up alternative paths to consider. This is only possible if the relationship is established and trust is gained.

Throughout your conversation, be aware of whether you are downloading, fact-checking, empathising or generativity listening. We are always aiming to make sure we are aware of how we are listening, and we want to inhabit that generative mindset where we are truly open to co-creating the therapeutic alliance with the person.

Here is a top 20 list of how to be an effective listener.

1. Set the scene.

   Before you start, make sure you have a welcoming and comfortable environment. Find a good chair, and make sure there are no other competing loud noises or quiet them down. Close the door if appropriate and ask the person if they feel comfortable.

2. Maintain eye contact with the speaker if possible.

   This is such an easy yet overlooked way to show someone you're engaged. It can be difficult with our current use of technology and taking notes during an interview, but make sure you use every opportunity to make direct eye contact.

3. Pay attention by attending to the person.

   Listen for things you can pick up that may make the experience better for the person or that may guide you into a generative space. If you are open to it, the person may even give you good ideas for their own treatment.

4. Find areas of interest.

   Shared experiences or ways to relate are often useful ways to start forming bonds. You may even use opposites (supporting a rival team) but as a way of demonstrating love of a sport, for instance. Let the person guide you.

5. Judge what they say, not how they say it.

   Be gracious in allowing others to find their own voice when telling a story. Allow for incorrect terminology and redundancy, and try to really sharpen your listening and identify what they are trying to tell you. If emotions come into it, show them that's okay and let them experience it. What does it tell you about their story?

6. Don't interrupt, and be patient.

   We've emphasised this many times, but keep yourself true to this. And if someone gives short, one-sentence answers, use phrases like 'Can you tell me more about that?' or 'What else would you say about that?' Use silence as your friend and give the person a chance to collect their thoughts as you move forward in the conversation.

7. Hold back your points or counterpoints.

Give the story some air, let it breathe and don't fall back to your own beliefs and experiences immediately. It may become important to share this later on, but initially, really listen and make sure you have their story the way they are intending it to be heard.

8. And what else?

When used skilfully, this question can be very powerful. Often people will hold something back, and this question is an invitation to think more deeply. You can also try, 'And what else have you tried?' or 'And what else do you think is contributing to the issue?'

9. Resist distractions.

No phones. No emails. No messages. As far as possible, try to create a space free of disruption and distractions.

10. Pay attention to nonverbal information.

This is important for you and the patient. Do they have their arms or legs crossed? Are they relaxed (shoulders, chest)? What is their breathing like – facial expression, eye contact? What are their hands doing? All these nonverbal cues might help to give even more richness to the words they are using. And think of your own nonverbal cues as well.

11. Keep your mind open and be adaptable.

It is important that you start the right way. If you're having a busy day, make a short list of things you might have to keep in the back of your mind. When you are with the person, let them continue to lead you into a deeper understanding of what their experience, beliefs and expectations might be.

12. Ask questions during pauses.

When there is an opportunity, facilitate the conversation with open and safe questions. If you need a moment to get your own words straight, do that. Keep these natural breaks in conversation for note-taking, and then continue with focused attention. Good questions will help clarify the main themes and create awareness of certain aspects.

13. Give feedback.

Tell the person what you are hearing, summarise key points and sense-check that with them. Use phrases like 'What I hear you saying is …' or 'Help me understand'. Paraphrase and use the feedback opportunity to discover what the person's true needs are.

14. Use yourself!

What comes up for you as you listen to the patient? Did what they said or did stir a particular response? Perhaps there is insight for both of you in that. Take time to share possible impressions but be careful not to make it about you.

15. Bring the conversation into the here and now.

It is really easy to talk at conceptual, abstract levels. But what does the information mean for us right now? Use phrases like 'What is going on right now for you as you say that?'

16. Present scenarios and options.

Rather than moving quickly to telling people what is wrong and what they need to do, offer situational context to your insights that enable the other person to apply things to their own world.

17. Reframe.

We often like to make judgements about the information as we see it. Reframing can be a powerful way to present a different perspective. Think of introducing ideas with 'What if you looked at it from this perspective?' or 'If that were to happen in this other setting, how would you respond?'

18. Make suggestions.

Suggestions are precisely that – they are not commands or expectations. Don't pressure the person to do what you suggest; simply offer an insight and invite the other person to pick it up. It's up to them.

19. Give advice and input.

There will be times when you have some important insight or knowledge that may help the person move forward. Think about how you might offer the advice in a way that the person is more likely to accept. What does it look like from their perspective? Address some of their potential concerns from the outset.

20. Provide challenge.

Just as in any high-quality interaction, there should be sufficient trust and safety to challenge well. Often patients will have incorrect assumptions or present inconsistent perspectives. Challenge with good questions; for example, if someone has been inconsistent in their approach, name what you have observed and simply ask, 'Why do you think that is?'

These are not meant to be a checklist for the listener, but rather tips that you need to incorporate in your listening and communicating with the person. Paying attention to these factors and developing these skills will allow you to get greater value, lean into the therapeutic alliance you're creating and give the person the best possible outcome.

Listening is not just the corralling of sounds, and certainly not a transcription of the words from a conversation. It is about connecting with the person in front of you, hearing their story and what it means to them and then exploring the best way in which this information helps to guide your involvement, in whichever way that may manifest. Sometimes that might take more than one session or emerge over time. Sometimes it may need silence, or rather not intervening straight away. By developing the skill of listening actively, generatively and with an openness for what that might lead to, you will move them into an unbreakable therapeutic alliance with your patients.

The entire interaction between you and the patient forms part of listening. It is about attending to the person, their needs and concerns, and really listening to their expectations, hopes and fears, understanding and beliefs. In that sense, you are in constant discourse with your patient, using your head, heart and gut to listen, allowing it to shape your responses and actions in a meaningful way. We are inviting our patients into this alliance and constantly paying attention to that relationship so that we may continue to grow together. Whether this is a single interaction or many years of multiple treatment sessions, listening allows us to gain meaningful insight from our patients and ourselves. It is a vital skill for the learning physiotherapist to move your practice into mastery.

Five Key Takeaways

1. Importance of listening: Clinicians often interrupt patients early into their explanation. This can hinder our attempts of building a trustful patient-clinician relationship. By listening carefully and not interrupting, we can understand a patient's self-obtained knowledge, experiences and perceptions about their condition, which can contribute to a foundation of trust.

2. The four types of listening: Otto Scharmer's four types of listening (downloading, factual, empathic and generative listening) highlight different ways in which a physiotherapist can interact with the information provided by the patient. Pay particular attention to generative listening – openness and a willingness to let go of preconceived ideas – as it is one of the most effective types of listening.

3. Role of facilitation and co-discovery: Rather than only providing information, physiotherapists should aim to facilitate a journey of discovery. This approach promotes self-awareness and responsibility in patients, leading to a greater willingness to embrace change.

4. Characteristics of good listening: Good listening is not just about silence; it involves active engagement, constructive questioning, providing feedback and creating a positive, supportive environment. Good listeners understand when to make suggestions and can adjust their approach based on the unique context of each patient.

5. Effective listening techniques: To be an effective listener, a clinician should create a comfortable environment, maintain eye contact, pay attention to nonverbal cues, keep an open mind, refrain from interrupting, resist distractions and ask probing questions during pauses. It's also important to give feedback, make use of personal responses, reframe perspectives, make suggestions, provide advice and, when necessary, provide respectful challenges.

Five Self-Directed Reflections

1. How can the dynamics of a clinical environment be changed to better accommodate different types of listening described by Otto Scharmer?
2. How do self-obtained patient knowledge and anecdotes influence the clinician-patient interaction and what strategies can clinicians use to navigate this?
3. How can clinicians incorporate behavioural learning in their practice to enhance the co-discovery process with their patients?
4. What are the potential barriers to adopting the four types of listening (downloading, factual, empathic and generative) in a clinical environment and how can these be overcome?
5. How can clinicians ensure they are practising generative listening during patient interactions, and what impact could this have on the therapeutic alliance?
Bonus: Conduct an interview with a patient or friend and record the interaction (with permission). Critically review the interview and determine where you use any of the 20 skills to be an effective listener detailed in the chapter. Then ask a colleague or a friend to do the same and see how many skills are identified by you and the other reviewer. Use this exercise to identify skills you are good at and those you need to develop further.

References

Alvey, S., & Barclay, K. (2007). The characteristics of dyadic trust in executive coaching. *Journal of Leadership Studies, 1*(1), 18–27.

Baron, L., & Morin, L. (2009). The coach-coachee relationship in executive coaching: A field study. *Human Resource Development Quarterly, 20*(1), 85–106.

Bordin, E. S. (1979). The generalizability of the psychoanalytic concept of the working alliance. *Psychotherapy: Theory, Research & Practice, 16*(3), 252.

Boyce, L. A., Jackson, R. J., & Neal, L. J. (2010). Building successful leadership coaching relationships: Examining impact of matching criteria in a leadership coaching program. *Journal of Management Development, 29*(10), 914–931.

Chester, E. C., Robinson, N. C., & Roberts, L. C. (2014). Opening clinical encounters in an adult musculoskeletal setting. *Manual Therapy, 19*(4), 306–310.

De Haan, E. (2012). Back to basics II: How the research on attachment and reflective-self function is relevant for coaches and consultants today. *International Coaching Psychology Review, 7*(2), 194–209.

Ferreira, P. H., Ferreira, M. L., Maher, C. G., Refshauge, K. M., Latimer, J., & Adams, R. D. (2013). The therapeutic alliance between clinicians and patients predicts outcome in chronic low back pain. *Physical Therapy, 93*(4), 470–478.

Fuentes, J., Armijo-Olivo, S., Funabashi, M., Miciak, M., Dick, B., Warren, S., Rashiq, S., Magee, D. J., & Gross, D. P. (2014). Enhanced therapeutic alliance modulates pain intensity and muscle pain sensitivity in patients with chronic low back pain: An experimental controlled study. *Physical Therapy, 94*(4), 477–489.

Gask, L., & Usherwood, T. (2002). ABC of psychological medicine: The consultation. *BMJ (Clinical research ed.), 324*(7353), 1567–1569. https://doi.org/10.1136/bmj.324.7353.1567.

Glueckauf, R. L. (1993). Use and misuse of assessment in rehabilitation: Getting back to the basics. In Glueckauf, R. L., Sechrest, L. B., Bond, G. R., & McDonel, E. C. (Eds.), *Improving assessment in rehabilitation and health* (pp. 135–155). SAGE Publications.

Gyllensten, K., & Palmer, S. (2007). The coaching relationship: An interpretative phenomenological analysis. *International Coaching Psychology Review, 2*(2), 168–177.

Hall, A. M., Ferreira, P. H., Maher, C. G., Latimer, J., & Ferreira, M. L. (2010). The influence of the therapist-patient relationship on treatment outcome in physical rehabilitation: A systematic review. *Physical Therapy, 90*(8), 1099–1110.

Heritage, J., & Robinson, J. D. (2006). The structure of patients' presenting concerns: Physicians' opening questions. *Health Communication, 19*(2), 89–102.

Horvath, A. O., & Greenberg, L. S. (1989). Development and validation of the working alliance inventory. *Journal of Counselling Psychology, 36*(2), 223.

Jowett, S., Yang, X., & Lorimer, R. (2012). The role of personality, empathy, and satisfaction with instruction within the context of the coach-athlete relationship. *International Journal of Coaching Science, 6*(2), 3–20.

Kaplan, S. H., Greenfield, S., & Ware, J. E., Jr (1989). Assessing the effects of physician-patient interactions on the outcomes of chronic disease. *Medical Care, 27*(3), S110–S127.

Lai, Y. L. M., & McDowell, A. (2016). Enhancing Evidence-Based Coaching Practice by Developing a Coaching Relationship Competency Framework. In L. van Zyl, M. Stander, A. Odendaal (Eds.), *Coaching Psychology: Meta-theoretical perspectives and applications in multicultural contexts (pp. 393–415).* Springer, Cham. https://doi.org/10.1007/978-3-319-31012-1_17.

Lee, Y. Y., & Lin, J. L. (2009). The effects of trust in physicians on self-efficacy, adherence and diabetes outcomes. *Social Science & Medicine, 68*(6), 1060–1068.

Lewin, K. (1951). *Field theory in social science: Selected theoretical papers.* (Edited by Dorwin Cartwright). Harpers.

Martin, D. J., Garske, J. P., & Davis, M. K. (2000). Relation of the therapeutic alliance with outcome and other variables: A meta-analytic review. *Journal of Consulting and Clinical Psychology, 68*(3), 438.

Nordquist, R. (2020). The definition of listening and how to do it well. ThoughtCo. https://www.thoughtco.com/listening-communication-term-1691247

O'Broin, A., & Palmer, S. (2006). The coach-client relationship and contributions made by the coach in improving coaching outcome. *The Coaching Psychologist, 2*(2), 16–20.

O'Keeffe, M., Cullinane, P., Hurley, J., Leahy, I., Bunzli, S., O'Sullivan, P. B., O'Sullivan, K. (2016). What influences patient-therapist interactions in musculoskeletal physical therapy? Qualitative systematic review and meta-synthesis. *Physical Therapy, 96*(5), 609–622.

Ong, L., de Haes, J., Hoos, A., & Lammes, F. B. (1995). Doctor-patient communication: A review of the literature. *Social Science & Medicine, 40*, 903.

Payton, O. D., Nelson, C. E., & Hobbs, M. S. (1998). Physical therapy patients' perceptions of their relationships with health care professionals. *Physiotherapy Theory and Practice, 14*(4), 211–221.

Pelham, G. (2015). *The coaching relationship in practice,* London: SAGE Publications. Available at http://digital.casalini.it/9781473942776 - Casalini id: 5018666.

Rogers, J. (2016). *Coaching skills: The definitive guide to being a coach.* Open University Press.

Scharmer, C. O. (2008). Uncovering the blind spot of leadership. *Leader to Leader, 2008*(52), 52–59.

Singh Ospina, N., Phillips, K. A., Rodriguez-Gutierrez, R., Castaneda-Guarderas, A., Gionfriddo, M. R., Branda, M. E., & Montori, V. M. (2019). Eliciting the patient's agenda-secondary analysis of recorded clinical encounters. *Journal of General Internal Medicine, 34*(1), 36–40.

Sonesh, S. C., Coultas, C. W., Lacerenza, C. N., Marlow, S. L., Benishek, L. E., & Salas, E. (2015). The power of coaching: A meta-analytic investigation. *Coaching: An International Journal of Theory, Research and Practice, 8*(2), 73–95.

Stewart, D., & Stasser, G. (1995). Expert role assignment and information sampling during collective recall and decision making. *Journal of Personality and Social Psychology, 69*(4), 619.

Sun, B. J., Deane, F. P., Crowe, T. P., Andresen, R., Oades, L., & Ciarrochi, J. (2013). A preliminary exploration of the working alliance and 'real relationship' in two coaching approaches with mental health workers. *International Coaching Psychology Review, 8*(2), 6–17.

van Dyk, N., Martoia, R., & O'Sullivan, K. (2019). First, do 'nothing' … and listen. *British Journal of Sports Medicine, July 1, 53*(13), 796–797.

Von Bertalanffy, L. (1969). General systems theory and psychiatry—an overview. *General Systems Theory and Psychiatry, 32*(4), 33–46.

Wampold, B. E. (2015). How important are the common factors in psychotherapy? An update. *World Psychiatry, 14*(3), 270–277.

Zenger, J., & Folkman, J. (2016). What great listeners actually do. *Harvard Business Review, July 14, 14.*

Zolnierek, K. B., & DiMatteo, M. R. (2009). Physician communication and patient adherence to treatment: A meta-analysis. *Medical Care, 47*(8), 826.

Zulman, D. M., Haverfield, M. C., Shaw, J. G., Brown-Johnson, C. G., Schwartz, R., Tierney, A. A., Zionts, D. L., Safaeinili, N., Fischer, M., Israni, S. T., & Asch, S. M. (2020). Practices to foster physician presence and connection with patients in the clinical encounter. *Journal of the American Medical Association, 323*(1), 70–81.

Further Reading

Elkins, D. N. (2007). Empirically supported treatments: The deconstruction of a myth. *Journal of Humanistic Psychology, 47*(4), 474–500.

Voss, C., & Raz, T. (2017). *Never split the difference*. Chicago, IL: Random House Business Books.

CHAPTER 5

Seeking Mentorship Consistently and Network Building

Colm Fuller ■ Marita Marshall ■ Steve Miller

> *'Master teachers and coaches don't stand in front; they stand alongside the individuals they're helping. They don't give long speeches; they deliver useful information in small, vivid chunks.'*
> – Daniel Coyle, consultant with MLB Team Cleveland Guardians and best-selling author of *The Talent Code* and *The Culture Code*

CHAPTER OUTLINE

Introduction	Prioritising Your Patients and Yourself
Core Values	Five Key Takeaways
Seeking Mentorship	Five Self-Directed Reflections

Introduction

The purpose of this chapter is to introduce the concepts of mentorship and networking, and to highlight the value of each.

Mentoring is often defined as the process of seeking external support to promote learning and growth by means of guidance and direction. It encourages clinicians to invest more in themselves by gaining a deeper appreciation of their own needs and goals. To get there, clinicians must pursue deeper levels of introspection, evaluation and reflection. As a process it can help clinicians take ownership of their career journey. An essential component involves building a professional support network, which provides the platform to seek guidance and generate opportunities, and thankfully, with technology, this has never been easier to do.

Networking involves building professional relationships and connections with individuals who can offer support, advice and potential opportunities for career advancement. It is the process of actively seeking out and nurturing relationships with people who have similar professional interests and goals. Effective networking involves establishing trust and rapport with others, communicating clearly and effectively and maintaining ongoing relationships. Networking can occur through various channels such as attending professional events, joining industry associations and utilising social media platforms. Building a strong network can be invaluable for career growth and development, as it can provide access to new knowledge, resources and opportunities.

> *'From an early age I knew that I wanted to work in the medical field. I was adamant that I wanted to work with people and not simply isolated behind a desk facing a screen. I was not clear on my exact career path but knew it would involve helping people.*

Now, not every situation will fit your career path but having a clear understanding of what you want makes it easier to begin the pursuit. Additionally, if you are having difficulty figuring out what you want to do, you may have already gathered some clues through identifying what you do not want. This information is hugely valuable as it will help you to wean out the opportunities which may be distractions from your pursuit and focus on the opportunities aligned with your dream career.'

– MARITA MASHALL, PHYSIOTHERAPIST AND FOUNDER OF IPOPS PHYSIOTHERAPY,
IN KNOWING AND UNDERSTANDING WHAT YOU WANT

Core Values

As introduced earlier in this book (see Chapter 2), understanding personal values is essential for achieving success in both personal and professional spheres.

Your core values will help maintain focus and align you with people, places, situations and things that drive your growth and career. If you are unsure of your core values, taking ownership of your self-awareness will allow you to reflect on your character and what you stand for. As per the exercises in Chapter 2, take a moment to note your core values, using the self-reflective questions and prompts.

By focusing on these questions, you can improve your understanding of your core values and enhance your self-awareness, ultimately contributing to your personal and professional success.

Seeking Mentorship

So, you have a clear understanding of what you want and know your core values. Perhaps you're a new graduate, an experienced physiotherapist or someone transitioning between roles or specialising in a specific domain of physiotherapy, but you're unsure about your next step in the field. Many can feel a sense of desperation when seeking desperation. It can be difficult to identify a starting point, despite reconigising that help is needed. I was not certain who to approach for guidance, but I knew I needed help.

Asking questions of those you admire and wish to emulate can offer valuable insights and perspectives that you wouldn't be able to access from an outsider's perspective. Being aware of your desires and core values can help you formulate the right questions to aid you in your quest. Thankfully, technology has made it much easier to connect with a diverse range of professionals at various levels of success. We propose an approach to mentorship that is focussed on three simple principles:

1. Show interest – this alone is enough to show your prospective mentor that they can afford time for you in the mentorship field.
2. Be ready to work – show and express willingness to learn and have a positive experience with your mentor.
3. Express gratitude – show appreciation for your mentor for taking the time to review your request.

BUILDING A STRONG NETWORK

Regardless of the stage of your career, a solid network can provide the extra confidence you need to overcome challenging days. It's essential to identify individuals and resources that can offer the necessary support at any point in your journey. This network may include educational resources, social media groups, professional associations, peers, journal subscriptions and YouTube pages. Once you've built your network, you should periodically re-evaluate its relevance.

Building a network requires intentionality and focus on your current needs.

LIFE CHANGES

As you progress through life and your career, your desires will evolve. What you want as an intern may differ significantly from your goals 5 or 20 years into your profession. Regular re-evaluation is crucial for staying committed to your present needs and setting the direction for your life and pursuits. By adapting to life changes and reassessing your network, you can ensure continued growth and success in your career.

> 'Growing up, I developed a fascination with people and their stories. I was exposed to many different cultures and backgrounds through family, travel, and a healthy social life. I learned how to connect with others, create a comfortable environment, and build relationships. Through introspection and learning from those around me, I began to understand the importance of different types of relationships. Although I never fully comprehended why some relationships were stronger than others or why I sometimes felt like an outsider in certain groups, I did recognise the importance of listening and learning from those around me.'

– COLM FULLER, HEAD OF PHYSIOTHERAPY, UPMC SPORTS SURGERY CLINIC,
IRELAND, IN *A LIVED EXPERIENCE*

WORLD EXPERIENCES

To build a strong mentoring network and advance your career, you need to gain diverse experiences and connections. This can be achieved by taking opportunities to travel, study and work in different countries, sectors and fields. By doing this, you will be exposed to new cultures, ways of learning and ways of working, which will help you expand your social and professional network, as well as your personal and professional growth.

It is important to recognise that your personal and professional network is not static, and it will change over time. As you gain more experience, some relationships may fade away, while others will become more valuable. Therefore, it is essential to maintain relationships with different people, such as friends, family, colleagues and mentors, as they can all provide different perspectives, insights and support for different problems.

It is also important to seek out academic and professional mentors who can provide guidance and feedback to help you achieve your goals. They can be instrumental in providing a sounding board for your ideas, giving you direction and opening doors for new opportunities. Mentors can also help you navigate through difficult decisions and provide valuable advice and encouragement. Often your academic mentors will have a significant influence on how you shape your personal life.

Finally, it is essential to challenge yourself and take on new projects that stretch your skills and expand your capabilities. Doing hard things will help you build confidence in your own work and learn new ways of expanding your skills, such as learning how to conduct academic research. It can also help you develop resilience, persistence and a willingness to take risks that can be invaluable for achieving your long-term goals. By putting it all together, you will be able to build a strong mentoring network and grow your career over time.

SUPPORT STRUCTURES AND ACTIVE REFLECTION

As a young clinician, you're likely to encounter challenges and setbacks in your career. Reflection can be a powerful tool to help you navigate these difficulties and learn from them. But to reflect effectively, you need a structure that allows you to engage in active self-examination and assess your values and purpose.

It's also important to recognise that reflection can be difficult and sometimes painful, especially when you're grappling with failures or missed opportunities. That's why having a support structure around you is critical. Seek out friends or colleagues who can offer honest and constructive feedback. They can help you validate your thoughts and offer empathy and perspective when you need it most.

Remember that feedback is not always positive, but it should be authentic and fair. Constructive criticism can be challenging to hear, but it's essential for growth. By actively seeking out feedback and being open to criticism, you can strengthen your relationships and learn from others.

As you build your mentoring network, keep in mind that different people can offer different types of support. Consider seeking out mentors who have expertise in different areas or who have had different career paths than your own. By expanding your network and seeking out diverse perspectives, you can broaden your horizons and grow both personally and professionally.

In summary, building a strong mentoring network requires active reflection, a support structure and a willingness to seek out feedback and learn from others. By engaging in these practices, you can navigate challenges and setbacks in your career and continue to grow and develop as a clinician.

> 'Most health professionals are empathetic and driven by a desire to help make a difference in the lives of others and gain a sense of fulfilment in doing so (I'm yet to find anyone driven by the financial rewards of healthcare delivery in the United Kingdom!).
>
> Many therapists may relate to being flexible with their time such as staying late to "squeeze" in clients, compiling rehabilitation programmes and running over sessions in their own time. As a result, the balance tips and important "me time" can slowly become sacrificed. This may include activities such as physical exercise (i.e., walks, runs or attending the gym) and social events, which can act as valuable stress-relievers and coping strategies.'

> – STEVE MILLER, PHYSIOTHERAPIST AND FOUNDER OF GROW PHYSIO, IN
> *CLINICIAN AND LIFE DEMANDS*

Prioritising Your Patients and Yourself

Rightfully, meeting the needs of the patient remains high up on the list of clinicians' priorities, but unfortunately this can slip into an unhealthy imbalance and even become an externalised focus and one-way process. Clinicians should give themselves permission to assign protected time to explore their own holistic wellbeing, generate new opportunities, manufacture new relationships, develop existing ones and draw upon the experiences and expertise of positive role models within their profession.

Health professionals are susceptible to self-sabotage. Inhospitable hours, demanding environments such as elite sport and the constant need to deliver for others can weigh heavily on clinicians.

Neglecting or devaluing your own needs may lead to future problems. Often, things do not surface until the latter 'crisis' stages before doing anything proactive about it, but it does not need to be this way. The key first stage is the realisation that clinicians too deserve a consistent, high-quality package of support, coaching and guidance. Visit Chapters 1 and 3 for practical ways to prioritise your self-care and wellbeing.

SO, WHO TAKES CARE OF THE CLINICIAN?

Clinicians need to prioritise their own wellbeing to effectively care for others. Mentorship offers significant benefits, not just for development but also in fostering resilience against work-related stress. It enables clinicians to understand and manage their workload better, to recognise when to take a break and to build confidence in setting boundaries. By investing in personal growth through mentoring, clinicians can enhance their capacity to meet professional demands, leading to improved patient care.

HOLISTIC CARE FOR PATIENTS AND THE THERAPIST

Mentoring can help avoid making these simple conclusions and help dig deeper into the needs of the person behind the apparent successes and ensure they are OK. It is OK not to be OK, and improving our understanding of ourselves is a high priority.

I HAVEN'T GOT TIME FOR MENTORING!

Most of us live full and busy lives! We juggle multiple balls within and outside of work, and working in healthcare often leads to us pedalling extremely hard and often leaves us feeling that there are not enough hours in the day. Naturally, this can limit the available time or headspace to consider what we personally want and struggle to see how we can strive to make life easier for ourselves and gain a better work-life balance.

It's commonplace to find ourselves trying to consistently satisfy patients, employers, colleagues and family needs. Subsequently, creating and protecting time to invest in ourselves can become rare. This precious time is typically one that is too easily sacrificed when things get busy.

SO, WHAT HAPPENS?

We often neglect self-care until we are overwhelmed. It is crucial to schedule regular 'wellbeing hours' for self-reflection and to engage with mentors for guidance. While finding time for this can be challenging and sometimes costly, it is vital. Your commitment to self-improvement, complemented by a mentor's support, can be key to advancing in your personal and professional life.

ACCOUNTABILITY

What drives you to complete a task or challenge? Is it anything to do with who you are accountable to? Is this an internal or external influence and does having that accountability help or hinder your progress?

Usually having accountability means we are more likely to be a 'finisher'. Some individuals have an ingrained drive and stick to to-do lists with commendable efficiency and consistency. However, most individuals complete tasks because of external pressures, deadlines and contractual and/or financial implications, which is understandable.

Once you set a goal, you may make a conscious plan on how you want to achieve it. Planning can be just the beginning of the journey, but starting, executing and finishing that plan is often the demanding bit and can benefit from a sounding board, checking in and evaluating progress and identifying whether you're coping with these demands or need pushing.

Motivation can come in waves. On a specific day you may be supercharged (usually with sleep and caffeine), raring to tackle the challenge head on. You may achieve a lot that day or you may be carrying out an essential stage of the journey that do not bring tangible benefits immediately. This can leave you feeling stagnant and demotivated; however, a good mentor can help steer you, reframe this and keep you on track.

REFRAMING, MOTIVATION AND STEERING

Whether the task in hand is focused on the next week, month or beyond, career aspirations, or your mental and physical wellbeing, it's proven to be more likely that you'll stick to it if you have someone to check in with periodically. This enables both parties to evaluate how far you have progressed and importantly to reflect on how the journey has been so far. Healthcare is a moving, evolving landscape and we need help from someone to embrace this change and potentially amend approaches or strategies to get to the end goal.

Everyone wants to see change/improvement regularly, but consider the ice cube melting analogy. At –5°C it remains ice; no changes are tangible at –4°C, –3°C, –2°C and –1°C until the temperature reaches 0°C, and eventually it begins to melt. Change comes with consistent engagement with the process. Elite athletes often reflect upon their success and highlight the process as the key focus point. Through self-reflection, we can improve our awareness of progress through process.

MAP AND MIRROR

A mentor serves two main functions: They help you to hold up a mirror to reflect your current self and a map to guide your future path. They not only assist in enhancing self-awareness but also in devising a plan for your aspirations. Unlike coaching or psychological therapy, mentorship is an interactive journey, relying on the mentor's insights to maintain your progress, even though the success of the journey ultimately depends on your own actions.

PICKING YOUR MENTOR

You need to have a mentor that you can believe in and can trust to steer you in the direction that you desire. They may or may not be an expert in your field. Certain personnel may provide this mentor role for no remuneration, but typically mentoring comes with some financial costs attached. Investing in yourself through mentoring is something that is starting to become more commonplace and can have a multidimensional effect on your wellbeing and career progression. Take David, an editor of this book … he counts amongst his mentors people like his Dad, Mike Davison (who wrote the foreword), Jay Hennessey of the Cleveland Guardians, RC Buford of the San Antonio Spurs, executive coach Tom Jordan, and his children Grace and Michael (his biggest teachers). Ciaran, also an editor, mentions the development of potential expert Fran O'Reilly, his Dad, older brother Seán, author and investor Alex Hormozi and Ray Dalio, who he doesn't know personally yet but has influenced his work profoundly.

I FEEL LIKE I'VE ACHIEVED SO MUCH IN MY JOB/CAREER BUT SOMETHING'S MISSING

Recognition at work often comes with increased responsibilities and rewards but this may steer you towards an unanticipated path. The challenge arises when these new responsibilities dictated by employers do not align with your personal goals, leading to potential discord between professional growth and personal objectives.

Consider the analogy of driftwood floating down a river. The river current will steer the wood down the stream, often at a predetermined rate, and the driftwood follows the path steered by this external current. This may be fine until the wood wants to change direction or reroute by doing its own thing. Unfortunately, if the current has become too powerful the wood may be stuck on a path it never intended to take. In healthcare or larger institutions there may be certain personalities or red tape that can be restrictive to an individual being creative or instilling change. Slow processes and reluctance to change may stunt personal development/growth, limit ideas and potentially bring feelings of frustration and resentment.

Subsequently, individuals can feel like they are not listened to, become disillusioned and lose motivation. Progressively this can leave employees feeling like just a number or a cog in a machine. Repeating this process over time may eventually cause an individual to lose sight of their own passions, transfer roles or even move jobs. Mentoring could help to better recognise and avoid this.

An opportunity to vent, feel listened to and be guided in a professional way could help generate positive change within the workplace.

CLINICAL SUPERVISION/APPRAISALS, COACHING VS MENTORING

From my experience, clinical supervision or annual appraisals are more about justifying that you're practising safely, that your notes are accurate and meet guidelines and that you can clinically reason and perhaps even learn a new manual therapy technique.

Don't be fooled: this is not mentoring! It often doesn't have your needs at the core, and it often feels like a tick-box exercise that helps prove that the organisation you work for is able to fulfil audit requirements in case governing bodies come knocking at the door.

But what if that person could 'mentor', support and help guide you to understand more about yourself and what you want to achieve so that you can outline a plan not solely to improve the patient experience (that will come naturally) but more about you as the clinician and what drives and motivates you?

AM I IN THE RIGHT PLACE CURRENTLY?

When you analyse yourself, you may realise that you don't appear to be in the right job, place or team at a particular time, which may limit your growth. It may be possible to manipulate your current role. Looking around you, surrounding yourself with the right people, environment and culture, can be crucial to enable you to grow and develop.

What if you never make this realisation? Familiar behavioural patterns are that you'll likely become resentful of the people and organisation around you. You may carry this burden into your personal life, affecting wider circles of friends and families. You may try to quash these feelings, but these negative connotations are likely to resurface and inevitably affect the quality of delivery to your patients/clients. Your characteristics, behaviours and personal 'brand' may gradually start to waiver and deteriorate.

YOUR JOB HAS TO WORK FOR YOU

Traditionally, jobs were solely a means of income and workers strived for higher salaries. In theory, higher salaries translate to a better life. However, as we move into a world of flexible hours, hybrid working and a greater appreciation of mental health and the wider wellbeing, money should just be one component when deciding on which job you deliver. It's important to remember that although you need the job, prospective employers need you and your valuable skill set and the additional qualities you bring to the team. Prior to starting a job is the time to negotiate because it is often much harder once you start, and contracts are drawn up and a mentor can help you understand the complexities, ask questions and guide you.

At times you may place your career at the forefront of decision-making, but how does this change with time or the introduction of family and wider responsibilities? Consider your ideal distribution and what you have currently. This will change throughout your life, and that's OK. Various categories such as work, family, friends and travel can all divide your time.

I WANT TO DO IT ALL!

Naturally, everyone wants to do everything, but we need to make choices. Often better skills, qualifications and money give you choices. Everyone will probably feel like a 'yes' man/woman at some point as they crave more opportunity, responsibility and recognition, but saying yes to everything is not always sustainable without losing out on social activities or burning out completely.

A mentor can help you realise what and where your values and passions lie and take stock of where you have distributed your beans or whether you can 'buy' some extra life beans or reclaim some if you have given them all away to others. There's a common phrase stating, 'Don't forget to fill up your own glass', pointing out that if you keep emptying your water into others' glasses to fill them up without refilling your own glass, you'll eventually have nothing left to give. Mentoring can help you gain perspective and self-help strategies that ensure you don't burn out, feel over-whelmed and eventually feel resentful towards others around you. Check in on yourself … if you were looking at your life as a friend would, what would you recommend?

'IT'S OK NOT TO BE OK'

It's also OK to not be sure why you're not OK, feel lost or feel that something's missing. A mentor can help with this, but a few questions are good starting points:
- What do you value most in your life right now?
- Why do you want to achieve what you want to achieve?
- How is your work-life balance? How are your beans distributed, and is this how you want them to be in the short-term vs longer term?
- How do you fill your own cup, and is this enough relative to how much you pour into others?
- What changes would you like to see in your life? What do you feel is hindering you the most from making those changes?
- Who are the most important people or things in your life, and what is your relationship to them, and do you allocate your time according to this list?

CELEBRATING SUCCESSES

- What are you most proud of in your life thus far? How did you achieve this?
- What previous steps have you already taken to achieve your goals? What has been the result so far, and what have you learned?
- Where do you see yourself (amount of time) from now? Is this where you want to be? Can you manufacture the necessary changes to get there? What do you think it will take to get there?

Overall, mentorship and networking are vital aspects to harness and create a lasting flywheel for success in physiotherapy. Not only do you receive feedback and clues as to where to focus your time from a mentor, but you also provide reciprocal value to an individual and build a mutually beneficial relationship along the way. Here are the key steps to take when seeking mentorship.

LOOK AT YOURSELF FIRST

Step One

Identify your own beliefs and list what your core values are. (See also Chapter 2).

These values are usually built over your lifetime from your experiences and your environment. They are engrained and are reflected in your personality, your communications, your thoughts and your actions. You may not like all of them or even see them in yourself easily, but through a process of introspection and self-assessment, identification of these core values will be very powerful for the development of your career. Conversations with close friends or family can help you to get input on how you tend to portray or demonstrate your beliefs to others.

Having strong beliefs can be extremely helpful to focus your attention. Beliefs drive behaviour. Beliefs affect your emotions. Beliefs can lead you into conflict or tricky situations. We know from pain science that strong beliefs can have a negative impact on your recovery.

Core values are definitively authentic. They should make sense to you and to everybody else. This is what you stand for. If you are on the fence, then that value is not core to who you are as a person.

Developing these values into a communicable commodity will give you confidence. It will allow you to shape your journey and identify with people who have similar values more easily. You will look for common ground because you will have more awareness of what you stand for and how to use that as a strength.

Step Two

Find your purpose and passion. It is essential to dedicate time and effort to this pursuit. Many medical doctors were previously qualified as physiotherapists. It is likely that they reflected on their career paths well before changing profession. Such reflections are critical, as they inform how mentoring should be approached, focussing on the true aspirations and goals of the mentees. You need to know what makes the other person tick and understand how they like to receive feedback. Understanding what mentees genuinely seek enables the creation of a supportive environment where they can openly discuss career apprehensions, facilitating impactful conversations that contribute to their personal and professional growth.

Step Three

Create some career goals. (See also Chapter 8)

These can change. Goals are not important for everything. Certainly, you cannot rely on motivation to get through a career. We hear regularly how discipline beats motivation every time. But setting some lofty goals can give you focus. Reach out to clinicians working at professional clubs, large organisations and even management roles in public and private healthcare. Seek opportunity to shadow. Offer your help and support and be willing to do hard yards. While working for no financial reward is not encouraged, it is also worthwhile considering the multiple benefits that can be acquired in subsidy.

The thought of working for free seems to be gone now. Unpaid internships that guarantee learning, development and accelerated career growth are no longer attractive. The benefit packages that are attractive nowadays have changed. This is important.

For mentors, it's important to change how young therapists view the world. It is important to understand that what worked in the past may no longer be attractive. However, the process of setting career goals can still really help. In fact, the answer is still the same. The goals should fit with your core values and your passion. That way, they will always be meaningful. They don't even have to be realistic right now. They should be audacious. They should be at the end of a long tunnel. You just need to create a network of support to show you the light.

Spending some time on your values, passion and goals should allow you to create a direction for your career.

LOOK AT WHAT YOU NEED TO SUPPORT YOU

Step Four

Get to know the person you think can be a mentor for you.

It is often helpful to see others in a strengths vs weaknesses comparison with yourself. What does this person have that I could get better at? How could this person's strengths embellish my own? This sounds ruthless at first. However, it is rarely done constructively and often just by subconscious osmosis. Your first step is to find common ground.

Build a social connection. Is this somebody that I recognise similar traits in? Is it somebody that might be interested in me and my story? How is their life interesting and what can I learn from it? Am I comfortable talking casually to this person and do I feel like I can ask silly questions? Do I have things that I can contribute to the conversation that will allow the potential mentor to get validation from helping me?

Of course, this all sounds quite intentional and there are few circumstances where you will need to consider this approach; perhaps when approaching somebody to be an academic supervisor, it fits the bill. But even then, your interactions with that person at the start of the relationship will dictate how it goes. You will need to be consistent with your messaging, be reliable when asked to perform tasks and force yourself to work hard to create a good impression. Then you will need to foster that and learn how to be consistent with that delivery.

Step Five

Identify your needs. (See Chapter 7)

Being reflective, you should have a fair idea of what you are good at and what you are not so good at. There are some things that you will just need to get better at. For example, in academia, learning how to store data securely and use statistical software are two important skills that require lots of practice and self-learning. A mentor can help you find the right platforms to learn on and which statistical tests to choose for analysis and review your work, but you will need to take ownership of the process and be clear on where you need help. You will also need to show progress in your learning. Develop principles to deal with weaknesses.

That process of reflection should allow you to identify what you really need:

- Emotional support
- Academic development
- Career progression
- Facilitating networking through introduction
- How to improve productivity and finish tasks
- Developing goals into actionable missions and constructing a pathway to get there

This will direct your conversations with your network and allow you to identify the type of mentor that will suit you best. Your connections will become clear, and your conversations will turn into growth opportunities.

Step Six

Build to last.

Going back to goal setting, your career direction will change several times. Situations will present themselves and that will allow your network to build and develop. Your interactions, both formal and informal, will continue to leave impressions on others and on yourself. Be conscious of the whole person, not just the clinician when giving support and feedback. Ask the question 'What way do you like feedback?' and give them a few options to help them answer it.

When seeking a mentor, understand that having mentors with different backgrounds will bring diversity in thinking and exposure to new experiences and ways of learning.

Of course, there comes a point where you have to make decisions, but it is far easier when you have clarity. And the longer that support group, mentorship, network or investment in you is there, the more valuable the input becomes. It starts to reflect who you are as a person, who you want to become and how you hold yourself accountable.

Some mentorships have no end point; they just change with the pressures of career development. If you get lucky, you can get lifelong support that will be more rewarding than any academic course, job or career path that you travel on.

Build your network to last.

Five Key Takeaways

1. It is important to identify your core values as they are ingrained in your personality, thoughts and actions and can affect your career development. Developing these values into a communicable commodity can give you confidence and help you identify with people who have similar values.

2. Finding your purpose or passion is important for your career. It can help you build your identity as a therapist, give you career-long focus and allow you to identify with and admire other people who have similar passions.

3. Creating some career goals can give you focus and direction, and they should fit with your core values and passion. They should be audacious and at the end of a long tunnel.

4. Finding a mentor can be helpful in seeing others in a strengths vs weaknesses comparison with yourself and can provide you with guidance and support in your career development.

5. Building a social connection with your mentor is important. Create a relationship that serves both participants and is one that lasts.

Five Self-Directed Reflections

1. How well do I understand my own core values, and how do they manifest in my actions and decisions?

2. What is my purpose or passion, and how does it align with my career path? Have I been able to identify it clearly, and if not, what steps can I take to discover it?

3. Have I set clear career goals that align with my core values and passion? How audacious are these goals, and what is my plan for achieving them?

4. How effectively have I sought out and utilised mentorship in my career? Have I consciously evaluated potential mentors based on their strengths and how they could complement my own?

5. How strong and mutually beneficial are my relationships with my mentors or potential mentors? How could I better foster these relationships to ensure they are long-lasting and impactful for both parties?

CHAPTER 6

Cohesive Working

Chris Morgan

> 'Without social cohesion, the human race wouldn't be here: we're not formidable
> enough to survive without the tactics, rules, and strategies that allow
> people to work together.'
> — Peter Guber, Chairman/CEO of Mandalay Entertainment and co-owner of the
> Golden State Warriors (NBA), LA Dodgers (MLB) and LA Football Club (MLS)

Introduction

Cohesive working is perhaps the most important factor in determining productivity and outcomes in workplaces for which a collective effort is vital to overall success. Given the interdependencies that exist in most modern organisations, team cohesion is a dynamic that needs to be actively worked on and not taken for granted.

In recent years, professional soccer has seen an explosion in the number of support staff in place to provide the perceived optimum environment for elite footballers to perform. When we consider how small the backroom staff was just 2 or 3 decades ago (less than 10 people) compared to the immense workforce that supports the modern athletes (around 100 people), the creation and nurturing of a cohesive working environment has never been more important.

The Individual vs the Group

The support network provided for individual athletes and the group as a collective is best considered the layers of an onion with the player at the centre. The layers are created through a combination of individual support (sourced and employed by the athlete), club support (identified and retained by the organisation) and coaching support (employed by the manager to deliver on their methodology and periodisation model). These multiple stakeholders, who have loyalties that lean slightly towards the player/club/manager depending on the employment background, are then tasked with the creation of a single support network for the group of athletes, which is simultaneously centred on the team and individualised to each athlete.

At its best, team cohesion works to amplify the skills and experiences of the individuals within the team. When not present, it does the opposite, suppressing the contributions of the individuals and resulting in a collective failure of the group and wider organisation. Quite simply, cohesive working should result in an outcome that is greater than the sum of its parts.

What It Is, What It Isn't

Cohesive working refers to a working environment where employees or team members work together effectively, support each other and have a shared sense of purpose. A cohesive working environment is characterised by open communication, trust and collaboration, which can lead to increased job satisfaction, higher productivity and improved results. Jonny Cooper, leadership coach and seven-time All-Ireland Gaelic Football champion with Dublin GAA, notes that a learning culture with strong cross-collaborative support fosters cohesion. He states that 'when people are connected to the higher purpose or the organisational goal' cohesion flourishes (Clancy & Dunne, 2020).

It is important to note that a cohesive working environment doesn't necessarily mean everyone has to be best friends or agree on everything. Rather, it is one in which people work together effectively and respect each other's differences. Professional conflict is a normal part of team cohesion – encouraging team members to engage in healthy debate without fear of offering an alternative opinion should be encouraged. In the past, this has been referred to as Psychological Safety (Edmondson, 2018). Similarly, in a previous role in an elite sporting organisation we spoke about 'rigour within, one message out', which actively encouraged the group to challenge each other in discussion phases, but to reach a relative consensus when it came to the collective decision of the group.

Building a cohesive working environment takes effort and deliberate actions from both employees and leadership, such as fostering a positive culture, encouraging teamwork and addressing conflicts in a constructive manner.

Meeting in the Middle

I have been fortunate to spend most of my professional career working in an elite football environment. As with most professional sports, football is hugely influenced by short-, medium- and long-term results, which often leads to a lack of coordination between subgroups of the organisation. As the group most affected by short-term results, the manager and coaching staff are likely to feel the tides of emotion associated with wins and losses the most. In contrast, club staff must balance the importance of the next result with the long-term plan and process for the continued evolution and success of the organisation. Thus, club staff must remain focused on vision and the organisational purpose, rather than getting swayed by every result.

These groups, of course, are not separate entities and will need to meet often in the middle to collaborate on short-, medium- and long-term planning. A good example of where this can seem to lack alignment is when a club makes a significant and obvious long-term investment in a new training ground. Such infrastructure is likely to be a part of the fabric of the club for the next 50 to 100 years; paradoxically, however, the club typically seeks the opinion of the manager and coaching staff, who are likely to be around for a very small percentage of the building's life.

Interdepartmental alignment and strong leadership are paramount for all individuals to feel valued and contributory to both the short-term goals and long-term vision of an organisation.

Even though football managers have a line manager who is responsible for making the decision on retaining or replacing them, when a club changes manager, it is as if the de facto leader of the entire club has been replaced. Certainly, in the UK, the team manager is seen as the overall leader for the vision of the club in terms of both playing style and culture. With this in mind and considering that managers change as often as every 18 months depending on the stability of the club, the vision and culture can change overnight and repeatedly. In organisations that have become toxic, this can be the perfect opportunity to implement change and improvement in team cohesion. In other instances, cohesive cultures can be wiped out by a significant change in key personnel and associated upheaval in leadership principles and behaviours. When you are on a journey towards cohesive working and success, you need to decide who you want on the bus, where everyone is sitting and who is behind the wheel.

Finding the Sweet Spot

I believe that there is a sweet spot in terms of the numbers who make up any team and that the sweet spot will be dependent on the environment, task and team culture. Clearly, no department wants to be understaffed to the extent that the sheer workload is not sustainable. However, it often feels that overstaffing is rarely the answer. So how do we know what the sweet spot is in order to maximise expertise, engagement, effectiveness and productivity with essentially the 'minimum effective dose'?

Google conducted an unpublished internal study to investigate what made their teams effective named Project Aristotle (Duhigg, 2016). Specifically, they identified similar traits in their most successful teams and collated information on what was important to various stakeholders. For those 'within' the team, the most important factors were the culture and the environment. Eventually they identified five key aspects that the best teams shared, as well as some things that made no difference (e.g., seniority, more people).

1. Psychological safety: where team members feel safe to take risks, be vulnerable and admit not knowing something in front of each other.
2. Dependability: where team members get things done on time and meet the organisation's high bar for excellence.
3. Structure/clarity: so that team members have clear roles, plans and goals.
4. Meaning: so that work is personally important to team members.
5. Impact: so that team members feel that their work matters and creates change.

These things are simple and quite intuitive, such that people want to feel safe, to be able to depend on teammates, to have clarity on what is expected of them and to do work that is both meaningful and impactful.

The landscape of professional football is in constant flux, with a lack of job stability and changing teammates creating uncertainty as to who is dependable. As alluded to previously, club structure is often altered in line with a new manager's vision, which leads to a lack of clarity. Similarly, an excessively large workforce with overlapping roles can cause people to feel so far away from the cutting edge of performance that their presence is meaningless. Being peripheral to both short- and long-term goals can leave someone feeling undervalued, unimportant and impactless.

The Building Blocks

To build a cohesive sports team, coaches and leaders (such as Sporting, Performance and Medical Directors) need to create a positive culture that values collaboration and teamwork. This can be achieved through artificial activities that build trust (e.g., team-building exercises) and open communication, but it is more likely to become the cultural norm when it is built by authentically celebrating the collective during times of success and avoiding the blaming of individuals during periods of failure.

It is important for leaders to address any conflicts or issues that may arise and to encourage all members of the group to work together and support each other. Additionally, a strong sense of team identity and shared vision contribute to a cohesive working environment, which can be achieved through clear messaging from leaders, team traditions and culture. When everyone is working towards a common goal that they have helped create, along with a plan that they have helped develop, they are more likely to support each other, overcome challenges together and perform at their best.

The best moments for any team are typically when all members are willing to take risks and be vulnerable, can identify excellence in their peers' work, have clear roles, goals and accountability, and, perhaps most importantly, appreciate their roles' meaning and impact.

Teamwork Makes the Dream Work

Ground-breaking work conducted by former professional rugby player Ben Darwin came to focus on the well-researched book *Edge* by Ben Lyttleton (2018). Darwin has researched *cohesion* and how great teams are more than just the sum of their parts. The research team with his company, Gain Line Analytics, believes great teams are formed by the linkages and connections within a high-performing organisation. This can, in turn, lend itself to more sustainable, long-term success, both in the sporting and business arenas. Cutting-edge evidence and real-world experience have helped form a unique metric, the Team Work Index (TWI®) – shared experiences, player combinations and the team system construct the TWI. Key Cohesion Markers are used to analyse the quantity and intensity of linkages within a team. The stronger the metrics, the more cohesive and 'well-gelled' the team.

Talent is rarely enough. Excellent management and coaching also. A group must be highly cohesive for sustained and consistent performance … and winning. As Darwin says, cohesion is driven from the top of the organisation down, from leadership. Without alignment, financial support and strong governance, cohesion can rarely be built and integrated across a performance system. Organisational design, talent benchmarking and recruitment processes can help significantly with this alignment process.

Row, Row, Row Your Boat

An analogy of a raft and a cruise liner is useful for understanding how leadership and collective team effort compare to a team of individuals who are just along for the ride.

Anybody who has ever been white-water rafting will know that the success of the trip is completely dependent on the teamwork of those in the raft, plus the leadership of the person steering from the back. Nobody can just come along for the ride. Those in the raft provide the energy to drive the vessel forward. Without that energy and teamwork, you can quickly find yourself in danger – heading for choppy water or a hidden boulder that can easily flip everyone out. The leader, similarly, is powerless if their crew is uncoordinated or unwilling and unable to work together.

A cruise liner is a contrasting experience entirely, such that the passengers are totally in the hands of the crew. They are essentially 'along for the ride', basking in comfort on a predetermined path. With all going well, the big cruise ship will gently pull into its destination without too much drama. The captain of the cruise liner is up on the bridge, while the rest of the people are down below, unable to communicate with the captain and his crew. If things do start to go wrong, however, it can take an age to turn the ship owing to the large numbers involved, most of whom are simply 'along for the ride', and the time it takes to recognise and act upon the danger.

Those in the raft will inevitably have a rougher ride, but they are vital to the journey's success. They need to be individually and collectively vigilant, alert, responsive and agile in order to enjoy the risk, support the leader and work as a team to safely reach the destination. They have a combination of role clarity and direct communication with the leader. It is clearly better to be part of a team that can ride the white water and do something about hitting that boulder, rather than isolated on a cruise ship as it hits an iceberg, with passengers staring out the window and commenting, 'I saw that coming'.

Workplace Benefits

Overall, cohesive working can lead to increased productivity because employees are better able to work together and support each other. A highly effective, cohesive working environment should look like a jigsaw puzzle with the strengths of the individuals recognised and utilised and weaknesses of the individual not affecting the group due to the strengths of others.

When employees work well together, they are more likely to collaborate effectively, share ideas and resources (thus avoiding the dreaded silos) and achieve better results. Open working spaces and shared breakout zones between different teams within an organisation are excellent ways for ideas to sprout and grow across departments. The environment that is characterised by open and effective communication will lead to improved understanding, problem-solving and decision-making while reducing conflict and disagreements.

A supportive and collaborative working environment will lead to higher levels of job satisfaction among employees as they feel valued and supported. It is often said that people do not leave organisations – they leave bosses. This shows the importance of creating an environment in which the individual feels valued and impactful within the organisation and in their work.

Is There a Downside?

Despite the overall positives associated with cohesive working, there is a tipping point where negatives can also start to become an issue.

Workplace cohesion can result in resistance to change, with some employees opposing a move away from the norm they have become comfortable with. This can be a big issue in professional football, as an example, where there is a danger that employees hang on to roles and, thus, are resistant to new ideas. They may also be resistant to new individuals who may destabilise the environment they have become accustomed to.

In a highly cohesive environment, a lack of individual autonomy can develop whereby the pressure to conform to the group results in the oppression of individual thought processes and ideas. Such an occurrence has a hugely negative impact on creativity and risk-taking. If allowed to prosper, this can further develop into 'groupthink', with employees far more likely to conform to the opinions and decisions of the group. As a result, healthy challenges and critical thinking diminish. In organisations involved in risk, this can have devastating implications. To mitigate this, it is crucial to involve new people along the pathway of decision-making who are more likely to question the process. A mentor can be hugely impactful in this 'check and challenge' approach.

As mentioned, psychological safety and professional conflict are healthy aspects of cohesive working, and a lack of disagreements should be seen as the early sign that the apparent cohesion is running into problems. An overly cohesive workplace can have difficulty in addressing conflict; conflicts may be swept under the rug or not dealt with effectively, leading to unresolved issues and tension. If people are unwilling to have difficult conversations, then corridor conversations and office gossip prevail, which may mark the beginning of the end for the cohesive environment that has been nurtured so carefully.

Finally, an overly cohesive environment can have difficulty accommodating diverse perspectives; it may not be able to effectively embrace diversity and difference, potentially leading to a lack of innovation and creativity. If you look around your team and see lots of people who look just like you, you are probably on the wrong team. Look for a team that embraces diversity and enjoys debate before reaching a common compromise, rather than one that glides alongside each other, agreeing for comfort.

A Final Word

While a cohesive working environment has many benefits, it is important to strike a balance between encouraging collaboration and support and maintaining autonomy and diversity of thought. It is vital that leaders address conflicts and disagreements effectively and spend time checking on individuals in a team to ensure that the work environment remains positive and productive. This is particularly important in the ever-evolving, voraciously competitive and fast-paced world of professional sport, where changing personnel and overlapping priorities between the individual and team require effective leadership and a highly cohesive working environment.

Five Key Takeaways

1. Building team cohesion in sports. For a sports team to excel, a culture that emphasises collaboration, open communication and collective celebration of success is crucial. Activities that build trust, along with addressing conflicts promptly, fostering team identity and establishing a shared vision, can contribute to a cohesive and high-performing team.
2. Understanding leadership and teamwork through analogies. The 'Raft vs Cruise Liner' analogy illustrates two contrasting styles of leadership and teamwork. Successful teams, similar to a well-coordinated rafting group, require clear roles, direct communication, vigilance and agility, with every member playing a crucial role in the team's success.
3. The power of cohesive working environments. Cohesion in the workplace enhances productivity, collaboration and overall job satisfaction. It allows for effective problem-solving and decision-making, and it reduces conflicts. However, cohesion shouldn't preclude professional conflict, as healthy debates can lead to better collective decisions.
4. Navigating the potential downsides of cohesion. While cohesion has many benefits, an overly cohesive environment can lead to resistance to change, suppression of individual thought and groupthink. Balancing cohesion with autonomy, encouraging diversity of thought and addressing conflicts effectively are key to maintaining a healthy work environment.
5. Balancing team structure and goals. In dynamic environments like professional sports, balancing short-term results with long-term vision is vital. Optimal team size and structure depend on multiple factors, including the task at hand and team culture. Effective leadership, psychological safety, clarity of roles and understanding the meaning and impact of individual roles are essential elements for team success.

Five Self-Directed Reflections

1. Do you consider team cohesion when it comes to recruitment and retention within your organisation?
2. Do you (and members of your team) have clear roles, responsibilities and accountability?
3. Are you able to identify the leaders of long-term, medium-term and short-term cohesion within your organisation?
4. How can you personally and collectively improve team cohesion in your organisation?
5. Are you on a cruise ship or in a raft? Describe how it feels.

References

Clancy, D., & Dunne, C. (Hosts). (2020, December 25). #100 with Jonny Cooper [Audio podcast episode]. In *Sleep Eat Perform Repeat*. Available at https://www.sleepeatperformrepeat.com. Accessed 7 March 2024.
Duhigg, C. (2016). What Google learned from its quest to build the perfect team. *The New York Times Magazine*. Available at https://www.nytimes.com/2016/02/28/magazine/what-google-learned-from-its-quest-to-build-the-perfect-team.html. Accessed 7 March 2024.
Edmondson, A. (2018). *The fearless organization: Creating psychological safety in the workplace for learning, innovation, and growth*. Hoboken, NJ: Wiley & Sons.
Lyttleton, B. (2018). *Leadership secrets from football's top thinkers: What business can learn from football*. London: Harper Collins.

Career Mapping

CHAPTER 7

Curiosity, Learning and Reflection

Kasper Thornton ▪ Paolo Policastri

> *'The challenges you face will test and strengthen you. If you're not failing,*
> *you're not pushing your limits, and if you're not pushing your limits,*
> *you're not maximising your potential ... Pain + Reflection = Progress.'*
> — Ray Dalio, philanthropist, Chairman of Bridgewater Associates, best-selling author of
> *Principles*, 2017

CHAPTER OUTLINE

Introduction

The world is in a state of constant change – and the field of physiotherapy and medicine is no exception to this trend. Every passing day brings forth fresh research papers, thought-provoking articles and an unending stream of informative podcasts. Furthermore, practical courses are being developed regularly, providing exciting opportunities for those seeking to expand their knowledge in this ever-evolving domain.

In this context, the ability to learn and develop continuously as a practitioner is becoming increasingly important. In this chapter we will discuss the importance of career-long learning and highlight motivations for doing it. These include personal growth, creating high performance and identifying one's passion. We will emphasise the power of knowledge and the various ways you can continue learning, including internships, shadowing colleagues and reading scientific papers.

Lastly, the chapter explores the technique of reflection and its benefits for professional development. By reflecting on past experiences, you can gain insights and improve your skills for the future!

The Importance of Career-Long Learning

The physiotherapy and medical professions are evolving faster than ever, bringing with them both opportunities and challenges. Because of the fast-paced nature of the industry, employees must keep up with the latest evidence and trends while working in high-demand jobs. Skills that were once required for a specific job may no longer be sufficient, emphasising the importance of continuing to learn and develop as a practitioner.

You will soon fall behind the curve if you do not continue to grow and develop. Successful practitioners place a strong emphasis on developing their own personal and professional skills, knowledge and talents to adapt to and prepare for shifting performance standards.

Consider this: We were encouraged to grow intellectually throughout adolescence, often with the phrase 'there's always room for improvement'. This should not be any different for you in your career. We must emphasise the importance of lifelong learning and development. Your future in the profession depends on it!

Top 10 Motivations for Career-Long Learning

1. **It's fun!**
   Everyone wants to learn – and we all would like to be better at what we do. You can choose freely between all of the many ways to better yourself and dive into the niches of the profession that you find the most interesting. You'll come to enjoy the process of learning and expanding your knowledge. The pleasure we derive from knowing and understanding is what makes learning fun.

2. **Personal growth:**
   This is one of the most important things you can have from career-long learning. With personal growth you can rely on many things; it's personal, but how can you grow without learning?

3. **It helps to create high performance:**
   By keeping up with the latest evidence and trends, you're more likely to become a high-performing individual. High performance is succeeding above and beyond standard norms, over the long term, while maintaining good mental health and overall wellbeing – a character trait that is highly sought after in today's job market.

4. **A competitive advantage:**
   Career-long learning will give you a competitive edge in the job market. Remember back in university. How many times have teachers had completely outdated slides? Look at today's social media and you'll see so much nonsense still being promoted. If you take the time and plan for your learning and education, this will definitely give you a competitive advantage in today's job market – and even more important, it will optimise outcomes for your patients. To plan for your development is to ensure you'll have high employability in the future.

5. **Having a dynamic life:**
   The term 'dynamic' can be linked to the concept of movement, which in turn implies being active. Being active can be summed up in the famous yet straightforward statement: 'live your life'. Therefore, a dynamic life is essentially an active life, and it is through movement that we can bring about positive changes, make improvements and gain new knowledge daily.

6. **Possibility to have a family:**
   Family means many things, not just a partner and children. If you rethink the competitive edge in the job market mentioned above, being more competitive means that you can economically improve, be ready to build a family, help your relatives or achieve whatever you set your mind to.

7. **Help to identify your passion:**
   Experience forms the path – use it to understand your personal growth and to find your passion. A profession is made up of several facets; many experiences drive many opportunities to find your favourite.

8. **Social growth:**
   Continued education is an important part of making the world a better place for everyone. Learning new skills will not only provide you with career opportunities but will also give you the chance to use the skills you have attained and give back to your community.

9. **Learning can be done in many ways:**
   Taking in new knowledge can be done in many ways – here are just a few examples of ways to keep learning throughout your career.
   - Internships.
   - Shadowing a colleague.
   - Take a trip abroad and see how the profession is run there.
   - Subscribe to your favourite publisher and make sure to plan time in your week to read scientific papers.
   - Follow evidence-based practitioners on social media. Twitter is a goldmine of knowledge when you know where to look and whom to follow.
   - Hone your skills with courses outside the area you normally work in. If you work in orthopaedics, make sure to keep learning skills outside that specialty.
10. **Knowledge is power:**
    Knowledge is power because it gives you the ability to make informed decisions, solve complex problems and develop new skills. It can help you to understand the world around you and make better decisions. Knowledge gives you the power to make the right choices and have a more successful life.

Why You Should Start a Deliberate Reflection Practice

Instead of doing things the same way you've always done them, reflecting allows you to improve your talents and assess their efficacy. It is about positively evaluating what you do and why you do it, and then determining whether there is a better or more efficient way to do it in the future.

Reflection is crucial to learning in any role, whether at home or at work. You wouldn't make a dish again if it didn't turn out the first time, would you? You'd either modify the recipe or come up with a new, presumably superior one. When we learn, we might become trapped in a habit that may or may not be productive. Thinking about your abilities might help you discover potential modifications.

A study on employees at a customer support centre who spent 15 minutes at the end of the day reflecting on lessons learned from that day did 23% better compared to those who did not when they were compared after 10 days (Di Stefano *et al.*, 2023). Likewise, a study of UK commuters revealed that individuals who were encouraged to use their travel to think about and organise their day were happier, more productive and less stressed than those who were not (Jachimowicz *et al.*, 2021).

Reflection as a System

Reflection is a process-oriented technique that allows you to obtain insight into your professional practice by analysing any aspect of it. The insights gained and lessons learned may be used to sustain good practice while also resulting in advances and improvements for both the professional and their service customers.

Various people learn in different ways, and while one person may learn best by reflecting on a great outcome, another may learn best by focusing on a difficult scenario. It is critical that you reflect on the method that works best for you to reap the most benefits.

Writing is widely used for reflection, presumably because it helps us to investigate and develop our thoughts more deliberately. It can, however, be in the form of a vocal sparring with a friend, colleague or mentor too. Consider 'adopting' the 5S Lean for reflection, developed by Hiroyuki Hirano in post-war Japan, where it was famously utilised by Toyota for leaner and better efficiency in their manufacturing facilities (Michalska & Szewieczek, 2007).

5S LEAN

The 5S Lean is a system used to improve efficiency, safety and orderliness in a workplace.

For a reflection practice this is how we can use it:

- **Sort** involves removing unnecessary items to reduce clutter.
- **Set** in order focuses on arranging essential items so they are accessible, to improve workflow.
- **Shine** is about maintaining a clean and tidy setting.
- **Standardise** establishes consistent procedures and schedules to help adhere to the first three steps.
- **Sustain** focuses on discipline and execution of the 5S principles to sustain over time.

Using a system such as this could improve productivity and quality.

How to Reflect

There are unlimited ways to reflect on your professional practices. On the simple end of things, you could take a moment every day, your 'reflection moment', which can be in the morning with a cup of coffee; it could be going for a walk or lying in bed before falling asleep – that could be your daily moment to think about the day and how to improve. This can be a good way to start your reflective practices, but if you really want to reap the benefits of reflections, you can go about it in a more structured manner, such as the 5 Whys, an iterative investigative technique. The 5 Whys strategy is a simple, effective tool for discovering the root cause of a problem (Fritze, 2016). It is often used in scenarios requiring problem-solving, decision-making and quality-improvement projects. Originating from Toyota in Japan, like the 5S, this is a system that could be engineered (pun intended!) for reflection hinges on posing the question 'Why?' five times.

Next we will focus deeper on the use of two specific reflection models: Borton's reflection model and Gibbs' reflective cycle.

Borton's Reflection Model

Borton's reflection model is a framework for reflection (Borton, 1970). Terry Borton, an American schoolteacher, created it in 1970. He described the approach in his book *Reach, Touch, and Teach*. He refers to it as the 'What, So What, Now What' style of reflective practice.

What: What has happened/what went bad/what went well?

So what: What was the outcome/what did you learn from the situation?

Now what: What do you need to do going forward? How do you improve?

And it really is as simple as that – it's asking yourself those three questions. Make it a habit to use this model on a daily/weekly basis and pick up on the small things that you think you could have handled better. Use the model to reflect on how to improve your outcome going forward.

Gibbs' Reflective Cycle

Another way of reflecting on your practice could be to use Gibbs' reflective cycle (Gibbs, 1988). Graham Gibbs created the Gibbs' reflective cycle in 1988 to systematise learning from events. It provides a framework for analysing events, and because it is cyclical, it lends itself particularly well to repeated encounters, allowing you to learn and prepare from things that went well or poorly. It is divided into six stages:

1. Description: Describe the situation or experience you've had.
2. Feelings: How did that make you feel? What did you think about it?

3. Evaluation: Evaluate how it all went – both the good and the bad.
4. Analysis: Try to make sense of the event; why did it happen?
5. Conclusion: What did you learn and what could you have done differently?
6. Action plan: How do you want to deal with the situation or experience in the future? How do you plan to improve your outcome?

Compared to Borton's model, Gibbs' cycle requires more time but also helps to provide even more depth to your reflective practice and might make you understand how you responded to a situation better. Where Borton's can be a model for daily reflections, Gibbs' cycle can be used on a greater scale to reflect on larger time periods or bigger events.

Curiosity Is a Superpower

In today's world, having a successful career means being able to stay ahead of the ever-evolving trends in the job market. Curiosity is one of the most important traits that can help any individual to achieve success in their career. It is the key to unlocking new possibilities and opportunities that are essential to staying ahead of the curve in an ever more competitive job market. Having a curious mindset is essential to staying ahead of the game and maintaining an advantage – no matter if you work in a hospital setting, in elite sports or in geriatrics.

Curiosity allows an individual to explore new ideas, concepts and technologies that will give them an edge over their peers, but more importantly, it will provide experiences and new learnings along the way. It is through the exploration of new ideas and technologies that one can stay up to date on the latest trends and developments in the ever-changing physiotherapy and medical industry.

Being curious also gives an individual a more open-minded outlook, which is essential for career success. An open-minded outlook can help an individual better understand the perspectives of their peers, patients and leaders. Curiosity is also essential for a successful career because it encourages creativity in problem-solving. Creative problem-solving is a highly sought-after skill and is essential for developing innovative solutions. By being curious and exploring new ideas, an individual can come up with creative solutions to complex problems, which can help them stand out from the competition – and help them solve the patients' problems more efficiently.

Finally, curiosity is a superpower because it encourages an individual to never stop learning. In a rapidly evolving job market, it is essential to have the skills and knowledge necessary to succeed. By being curious and exploring new ideas, an individual can stay up to date on the latest evidence, trends and technologies and be prepared for the ever-changing and fast-paced industry.

Overall, curiosity is one of the most important traits for career success. Curiosity is essential for unlocking new possibilities and opportunities that are vital for success. Curiosity is a superpower that can help any individual achieve success in their chosen career.

Five Key Takeaways

1. You must engage in career-long learning to succeed in the evolving physiotherapy and medical professions. To adapt to shifting performance standards, it's crucial to keep up with the latest evidence and trends.
2. Continuing to learn and continuing to develop your personal and professional skills and knowledge will be essential for your overall growth. This can help you create higher performance and gain a competitive advantage in the job market.
3. You can learn in many ways, including internships, shadowing, trips abroad, reading scientific papers, following evidence-based practitioners on social media and honing skills with courses outside your specialty.

4. Reflection is a valuable technique that allows you to gain insight into your professional practice. By analysing any aspect of it, you can sustain good practice and make advances and improvements for both you and your patients.
5. Knowledge is power, and having knowledge gives you the ability to make informed decisions, solve complex problems and develop new skills. Ultimately, this leads to a more successful career and maybe even a more successful life.

Five Self-Directed Reflections

1. How have you been implementing continuous learning in your career? What are some specific examples of skills or knowledge you have gained through this process?
2. What motivates you to continue learning in this profession? How can you leverage these motivations to facilitate more effective learning?
3. Reflecting on your experiences, can you identify a situation where continuous learning had a direct positive impact on your performance or outcome?
4. How have you utilised reflection in your professional growth? Which reflection model (Borton's or Gibbs') resonates more with your personal style of reflection, and how can you incorporate this model into your regular practice?
5. In what ways has your curiosity served as a superpower in your career? Can you recall instances where your curiosity led to creative problem-solving or innovative solutions?

References

Borton, T. (1970). *Reach, touch, and teach*. McGraw Hill.

Dalio, R. (2017). *Principles*. Simon and Schuster.

Di Stefano, G., Gino, F., Pisano, G. P., & Staats, B. R. (2023). Learning by thinking: How reflection can spur progress along the learning curve. *Management Science*. Harvard Business School NOM Unit Working Paper No. 14-093.

Fritze, C. (2016). *The Toyota production system. The key elements and the role of Kaizen within the system*. January 2016, pp. 1-13.

Gibbs, G. (1988). *Learning by doing: A guide to teaching and learning methods*. Further Education Unit.

Jachimowicz, J. M., Cunningham, J. L., Staats, B. R., Gino, F., & Menges, J. I. (2021). Between home and work: Commuting as an opportunity for role transitions. *Organization Science, 32*(1), 64–85. https://doi.org/10.1287/orsc.2020.1370.

Michalska, J., & Szewieczek, D. (2007). The 5S methodology as a tool for improving the organization. *Journal of Achievements in Materials and Manufacturing Engineering, 24*(2), 211–214.

CHAPTER 8

Goals and Motivation

Chris Desmond ▪ Filippo Siragusa

'Believe in yourself. Know that there is something inside you that is greater than any obstacle.'

— Rich Froning, winner of four consecutive CrossFit Games men's titles (Fittest Man on Earth) and winner of multiple team titles with CrossFit Mayhem

CHAPTER OUTLINE

Introduction

What Stands in the Way of Fulfilment?

Understanding Motivation

Understanding Your Inherent Motivations

Goal Setting in Physiotherapy

Five Key Takeaways

Five Self-Directed Reflections

Introduction

The aim of this chapter is to assist you in pursuing a fulfilling career as a physiotherapist in the context of a fulfilling life.

A career as a physiotherapist is by no means easy. In a 2019 workforce report commissioned by Physiotherapy New Zealand, almost 30% of respondents had left or were planning on leaving the profession. Of the respondents who indicated that they were not planning to leave the profession, one-fifth stated they would take a non-physiotherapy job at the same pay rate (Reid & Dixon, 2018).

Physiotherapists work in high-pressure environments with people who are facing some of the most challenging times of their lives. The support we get to provide is both rewarding and demanding. Alongside physiotherapists leaving the profession, we also experience high levels of work-related stress (Carmona-Barrientos *et al.*, 2020; González-Sánchez *et al.*, 2017).

Despite negative statistics, a career as a physiotherapist can be extremely fulfilling, as evidenced by the case studies in this chapter and the physiotherapy role models that you hopefully see in your communities.

Just like creating a rehabilitation program with a patient, the most fulfilling career results are achieved when your plan is individualised to you and your life context. The key to unlocking your sustainable fulfilling career is understanding your individual motivations and then selecting opportunities and setting goals that align with them.

What Stands in the Way of Fulfilment?

When it comes to understanding our individual motivations and seeking opportunities that align with them, there are often professional barriers.

In their 2018 book *Dark horse: achieving success through the pursuit of fulfillment*, Todd Rose and Ogi Ogas, researchers from Harvard University, argue that the standardisation of educational institutions and organisational practices does little to support the ability of the individual to understand and express themselves. Instead of unlocking the potential of individuals, educational institutions attempt to create outputs that can fill a certain job role – in this instance, a physiotherapist. Organisations also operate from standardised practices, utilising people to fill a particular role and then replacing them with another when they leave. The job shapes the people, rather than the people shaping the job.

In the context of physiotherapy, our university curriculums are developed in accordance with strict criteria from qualifications and regulatory authorities. While we have fantastic teachers through university who challenge us to grow in many ways, the desired outcome of our degree is to produce a physiotherapist who is safe and competent to practice.

Safety and competence are absolute necessities for our practice. Perhaps as well as the clinical reflective practice we perform, developing personal reflective practice should be emphasised just as strongly. There are examples of universities that are beginning to assist people to develop as well as produce physiotherapists. Hopefully, individualisation can sit alongside standardisation in the future of physiotherapy education.

Following university, we enter the workforce and the challenge of standardisation once again impacts the development of personal fulfilment. Each country has its own regulatory body which sets out its standards of practice. In many countries, physiotherapy treatment is funded or partially funded by insurance companies or governments. The rules and incentives that the regulatory bodies and funding providers set out inform the practice of physiotherapy. These rules are created for the safety of both physiotherapists and clients and to encourage efficient 'best practice' physiotherapy in the case of funders.

The organisations that we work for are constrained or incentivised by these rules. Rather than supporting our individual career, these incentives are instead created to deliver a standard product of physiotherapy. We again find amazing managers or mentors in workplaces, just like our teachers at university. However, these managers and mentors have developed within the constraints of the healthcare system and face the same challenges as us. Additionally, many of them do not have the skillset or the capacity to assist us to develop our individual career.

If we want to lead a fulfilling career as a physiotherapist, the onus falls on us to develop that. To do that successfully requires a deep understanding of our unique motivations and, subsequently, strategies to pursue them.

As individuals we are uniquely motivated. No two physiotherapists will have the same array of motivations. Yet many of us will follow a version of the standard physiotherapy career pathway rather than understanding our drivers and pursuing opportunities in alignment with them.

Much motivation research within the physiotherapy profession focuses on external motivating factors. These are factors like remuneration, peer support, autonomy of practice and recognition (Latzke *et al.*, 2021). The majority of these motivating factors sit outside of our sphere of control (Covey & Covey, 2020). We have little to no agency over them other than hoping that the opportunities we pursue will provide them.

The patients, clients and athletes we work with are all unique. They require an individualised approach to their rehabilitation to achieve results that are meaningful to them. Just like the people we work with, we also require an individualised approach to our careers to ensure they are meaningful and fulfilling.

Understanding Motivation

We each have a unique array of motivations (Rose *et al.*, 2013). However, these motivations can be categorised into three broad categories. Each type of motivation is valuable and has been shown to have variable effects on our persistence and performance levels in the workplace (Grant, 2008).

INTRINSIC MOTIVATION

Intrinsic motivation is the 'doing of an activity for its inherent satisfaction rather than for some separable consequence' (Ryan & Deci, 2000, p. 56). When we are intrinsically motivated, we enjoy an activity for the activity's sake; performing it gives us a 'twinkle in our eye'. These activities may or may not lead to an external outcome. Regardless of this outcome we would do them anyway. Intrinsic motivation has been shown to be positively associated with persistence and performance, especially when coupled with prosocial motivation (Grant, 2008).

Little children are very intrinsically motivated – they love to play and to learn. They are drawn to activities they enjoy. In turn, they are active, curious and eager to engage their environments, and when they do, they learn. To some extent adults also love to play and to learn. Throughout life, when they are in their healthiest states, adults are active and interested, and the intrinsically motivated behaviours that result help them acquire knowledge about themselves and their world (Ryan & Deci, 2000).

The construct of intrinsic motivation describes the inclination towards assimilation, mastery, spontaneous interest and exploration that is a principal source of enjoyment and vitality throughout life (Ryan, 1995).

PROSOCIAL MOTIVATION

Prosocial motivation describes the desire to benefit others or expend effort for others. Prosocial motivation drives action with the intention of helping others. This motivation occurs most strongly when the 'others' in question are those we care about or are similar to us in some way. It is more difficult to feel motivation to assist someone to whom we do not relate. This is the motivation to get a gift for a loved one to see their enjoyment or to donate time or money for a cause that you care deeply about (Grant & Berg, 2012).

This type of motivation is positively associated with persistence and performance, with its effect size increased when coupled with intrinsic motivation (Grant, 2008). Prosocial motivation has also been shown to increase our ability to be creative and solve problems (Grant & Berry, 2011; Tian et al., 2021), skills required when creating a fulfilling career for ourselves.

EXTRINSIC MOTIVATION

Extrinsic motivation describes behaviour occurring in anticipation of an external outcome. This is when we do the work to reap the reward or to avoid the punishment not doing the work entails.

Extrinsic motivation is often considered the weakest form of motivation when it comes to persistence and performance (Grant, 2008). We are less likely to persist with an activity if we do not find it inherently satisfying and it does not benefit others we care about. At times pursuing extrinsic motivation can be counterproductive to creating a fulfilling career. Selecting opportunities based on extrinsic rewards that don't also align with our values creates cognitive dissonance. Mental and emotional discomfort occurs when our actions do not match our values. Physiotherapy offers many opportunities to pursue extrinsic motivators. These include certifications and degrees, pay rises and other forms of recognition and authoring academic papers or in this instance textbook chapters. However, extrinsic motivation is not necessarily counterproductive to fulfilment (Ryan & Deci, 2000). Certifications, recognition and publications can and do add to our enjoyment of life. For the most part I've thoroughly enjoyed writing this chapter.

To select more fulfilling opportunities, we need to look more closely at the facets of extrinsic motivation. Self-determination theory describes extrinsic motivation through four different regulatory pathways.

External Regulation

Externally regulated behaviours are performed in order to satisfy an external demand or reward contingency. These behaviours are performed to be compliant with a set of rules and to achieve a reward or avoid a punishment associated with a consequence of those rules. Actions are performed because of a perceived external locus of control.

Introjected Regulation

Introjected behaviours involve taking on a regulation but not fully accepting it as one's own. Behaviours are performed to avoid anxiety or guilt or attain ego enhancements such as pride. This type of motivation is associated with feelings of self-worth. These behaviours are internally driven but still have a perceived external locus of control.

Identified Regulation

Identified regulation describes a conscious valuing of a behavioural goal in a way that the action performed is accepted or owned as personally important.

Integrated Regulation

Integrated regulation occurs when behaviours are fully assimilated into the self. They have been evaluated and are in congruence with your other values and needs. Integrated regulation has many similarities to intrinsic motivation; however, they are still considered extrinsic as they are performed to obtain outcomes rather than for inherent enjoyment (Ryan & Deci, 2000).

We can view identified and integrated regulation as motivation inherent to ourselves. This motivation contributes to fulfilment (Ryan & Deci, 2000). These behaviours contribute to supporting our values and have an external outcome attached. They may improve our self-esteem or status in the eyes of our peers but as a byproduct of our behaviours rather than as motivations in themselves.

Along with identified and integrated regulation, intrinsic and prosocial motivation are inherent to each of us. When we understand and act in accordance with our inherent motivations, it manifests as enhanced performance, increased persistence (Deci & Ryan, 1991; Grant, 2008; Sheldon *et al.*, 1997), increased creativity (Tian *et al.*, 2021), heightened vitality (Nix *et al.*, 1999), self-esteem (Deci & Ryan, 1995) and wellbeing (Ryan *et al.*, 1995).

Your motives comprise the emotional core of your individuality. What you desire and what you do not define who you are in a unique and personal manner. When you act and pursue opportunities congruent with your individuality, it reduces dissonance and increases fulfilment.

Understanding Your Inherent Motivations

As you define your inherent motivations, resist the sense that you 'should' be motivated by universal motives. Following universal motives places you at risk of overlooking your own. Just because everyone else is doing it doesn't mean that you should as well. A 'standard' career pathway based on the motivation of helping people risks overlooking your individuality.

Your thinking and understanding will evolve over time. The process of understanding your inherent motivations is an infinite game (Carse, 2011); there is no end to it. You will understand yourself more deeply over time. You will also evolve as you experience new things, consume more knowledge and interact with a quickly changing world. There is no end point to growth and self-awareness.

Rose & Ogas (2018) suggest a three-step process to assist in identifying your inherent motivations that they call 'the game of judgement'. The aim of playing the game of judgement is to use your instinctive reaction to others to identify the emotions behind the reactions and attempt to trace them to their source.

First, become aware of moments when you are judging someone. This is something we all do all the time. It's human nature to react to others, whether a patient, manager, partner, store clerk or our local barista. While not projecting judgement is beneficial in our clinical practice, we need to consciously attend to the times we do have a judgement reaction.

Second, identify the feelings that emerge as you reflexively judge someone. Vivid reactions indicate a strength of feeling, which leads us to our motivations and values. It doesn't matter whether the reaction is positive or negative if the feeling is pronounced. Try to identify the emotions that occur with the reaction. It's tempting to stop after identifying one strong emotion; however, on closer inspection there is often a constellation of emotions occurring simultaneously. I personally find an emotion wheel a helpful tool for this step of the process.

And third, ask yourself why you are experiencing those feelings. Be honest with yourself. Just like when we stop after identifying one emotion, our temptation is to stop analysis at the first answer. Rarely does this create genuine awareness of our motives; often it is a convenient answer we have not thought deeply about. To counter this tendency, adopt a strategy created by Sakichi Toyoda called the '5 Whys'. After answering the first 'why', respond to the answer you give with a further question, 'Why?' Repeat this process five times and it is likely you will be close to understanding the root motivations and the nuances contained within them.

Understand that you do not just hold one motivator but a range of different motivators, and it is important to identify and understand the full range to create a fulfilling career.

APPLY YOUR INHERENT MOTIVATIONS

Once you are aware of your inherent motivations, it is important to ensure that you seek out and decide on opportunities that align with these motivations.

The key to creating a fulfilling career is not always following the one motive that burns the hottest, but it is also in leveraging as many different motivators as possible. When selecting opportunities, look for the ones that provide the best fit for your unique motives. Rose & Ogas (2018) say to always look for opportunities with a better fit. They suggest pursuing better-fitting opportunities if you can live with the worst-case scenario, as small differences in fit with your motives can lead to large differences in fulfilment. This does not necessarily mean jumping from one job to the next. Opportunities can be created in the current role you occupy. In one of my previous roles, I arranged to help the marketing team with their content development so that I could satisfy my creative motivation. Once you understand your range of motivators it becomes easier to identify opportunities that you may have missed if you were focused on the 'standard' physiotherapy career pathway.

Outside of your inherent motivations there are other considerations when selecting opportunities to pursue. Opportunities that provide us with competence, autonomy and relatedness are more likely to lead to fulfilment and satisfaction (Deci & Ryan, 1995). Competence is to gain mastery of tasks and learn different skills. When we feel that we have the skills needed for success, we are more likely to take actions that will help us achieve our goals. Autonomy refers to our ability to exercise choice and a feeling of agency over our behaviours. Relatedness involves feelings of belonging, actually enjoying the people around you and the culture associated with the work. These themes were backed up by a Latzke et al. (2021) study of physiotherapists' job satisfaction in Austria. These physiotherapists identified that autonomy, recognition and social connectedness opportunities were strongly related to job satisfaction.

Understanding your range of motivations and being able to select opportunities that fit, which also supply competence, autonomy and relatedness, is the beginning. Selecting goals creates action towards a career of fulfilment.

Goal Setting in Physiotherapy

WHAT IS GOAL SETTING?

The Oxford English Dictionary defines a goal as 'the object to which effort or ambition is directed; the destination of a (more or less laborious) journey. An end or result towards which behaviour is consciously or unconsciously directed' (Wade, 2009, pp. 291–295).

Goal setting (GS), and consequently sharing a goal with a patient, is a key component of modern rehabilitation. It has been recognised as a valid tool to enhance the management in terms of adherence and share a patient-centred attitude (Stevens *et al.*, 2017) of chronic conditions (such as low back pain) in clinical rehab (Coppack *et al.*, 2012).

'Start with the end in mind' (Chia *et al.*, 2022) is a model of GS that is nowadays widely proposed in high-performance environments and rehab settings. It requires backwards design skills, which can facilitate physiotherapists to work backwards logically and intentionally to design transferable and context-specific rehabilitation plans that improve sports injury rehabilitation practices.

This includes the first step of defining a performance goal that includes a needs analysis of the sports in the context and then determining the key performance indicators (KPIs) and technical goals of the rehab process, the assessment of the current level of performance or restriction of the athlete the planning of the rehab process. Also, Dekker *et al.* (2020) proposed a practical model that would take into consideration the exploration of meaningful beliefs, attitudes and aims, putting together a program towards a client's overall goal and setting specific 'smaller' milestones to achieve the overall goal.

GS is surely a well-known practice and quality standard in the development of the professionalism of a physiotherapist (Bulley *et al.*, 2004). GS can rely on the development and the planification of a theoretical and practical framework that would focus mainly on self-efficacy, dealing with expectations and beliefs, taking a plan of action and how to adhere to it and feedback on the progress towards the goal set (Scobbie *et al.*, 2011).

Even if, as professionals, we are familiar with this approach, building a professional identity in physiotherapy can be a complex process to determine and program (Hammond *et al.*, 2016).

Hammond *et al.* (2016) define professional identity as a highly personal and dynamic process since it can include the career's moments, situations, experiences, attributes, beliefs, motivation and other contingencies that can lead to reinterpreting the professional self-concept. Also, family aspirations and the balance between work and private life can play a role (Mazerolle *et al.*, 2015) and be considered significant variables of a life/work story, as much as other pragmatic aspects of a workplace such as boundaries and hierarchies, mentorships and so on.

The trajectory of a career can show different and variable aims and expectations depending on the experiences made. Survey research proposed by Øster *et al.* (2017) explored the expectations of newly recruited physiotherapists in Europe and a meaningful result was defined as 'dreaming of making a difference/having an impact' and exploring the variety and the possibilities given by the profession. Naturally these statements can be considered relevant for a certain period of the career but could slightly lose importance through professional and personal development.

Whatever we consider a patient-centred approach or a personal/professional approach, GS is often combined and shared with a multidisciplinary team that has a commitment towards a meaningful outcome. This should be particularly clear working in high-performance medical staff (Salcinovic *et al.*, 2022), where the ability to set meaningful goals can be particularly important working in high performance medical staff.

The basic idea should consider GS in professional development, highly customised and directed by different variables. These can include physiological (quite primary), psychological, pragmatical, passional, self-esteem and self-actualisation issues.

Concretely we can consider the process of GS as the opportunity to increase an aspect of interest, realise something, improve or simplify something and develop yourself as a person and as a professional.

HOW CAN WE SET GOALS?

Goals should be intrinsically motivating first of all and have a personal dimension and value. Then they should be set for the person, respecting basic and personal factors such as lifestyle and aspirations and only limited by the presence of external factors or sources.

One of the first key focuses in setting our professional goals surely relies on the awareness of our values as individuals and therefore which values lead to the professional goal that we want to achieve.

A few common acronyms have been suggested to build up your GS mechanism, and all mainly converge on the definition of the level of clarity, challenge, commitment and complexity (not too easy, not too hard) of the goal, and a system of feedback over your actual progress towards the goal.

SMART(ER) goals can be considered a good methodological entry-level, basic approach to set your goals in your professional career, aware that the project and work-life balance considerations can lead to different decisions depending on individuals in certain moments of life. Also, different levels of motivation can interfere (not necessarily in a negative way) with personal priorities and importance, considering how family life and working career can change pretty suddenly.

SMART(ER) can have a few different declinations but generally stands for:

- **S**pecific to the process you want to take part in. Giving a 'where' and 'when' – avoid vague goals, for example 'within December I want to get all the requirements for a certain job and apply'. Other attachments can be stimulating, significant, simple and so on. At this step, you should ask yourself the details of your purpose, what you think it will take to be accomplished and the actions you are going to take and why you consider it relevant. This effort should lead to trying to go beyond superficial considerations or those imposed by others, since it can be quite common in academic and working environments to say 'I have to' or 'I need something for an advancement or promotion' (University of California, 2017). This is also a mature moment of self-awareness exploration, where you should carefully consider the aspects that can be related to the individuals involved in your plans and how to involve them in the accomplishment of the goal (the most involved are family, colleagues, friends, mentors and contacts).
- **M**eaningful to you (some other guidelines would use measurable, but it is more technical than job-oriented) and not to try to please other people. Also be aware of giving a certain level of complexity since a goal presented as too easy would probably lose the sense of meaning.
- **A**chievable (other terms used: attainable, acceptable), not going beyond what's a true expectation (even unrealistic). Surely your goal should inspire you to get to work and learn new skills, mindsets or different behaviours that can lead you to the discovery of something meaningful.
- **R**elevant (other terms used: rewarding or reasonable) to you. First of all, you should be sure with yourself and have awareness of the compatibility of your goals with the commitment required. Try to be honest and understand if your goals can be tolerated with other key aspects of your life. Once again, aspects such as family, obligation, personal health and wellbeing are all factors that should be taken into consideration.

TABLE 8.1 ■ Goal Setting Matrix

Goal	Real-world definition	Turn into SMART(ER)	Example of practical achievement that can help	Barriers and facilitators
I want to ….				

- **T**ime-bound, reinforcing the specificity of your goals by setting deadlines and moments of feedback. This works as a frame and a panoramic view of the duration of your intention. Further, and more practically, this helps give you priorities and urgencies relative to real-life barriers.
- **E**thical. As professionals, working with the health, expectations and education of the people we care for, we consider this as a key added value; therefore, an ethical goal in line with the deontological profile of the physiotherapist and your own morals and principles should be implemented. Note the importance of setting goals for what is meaningful for the patients (World Physiotherapy Association, n.d.).
- **R**ecorded. Another added value can be brought by the physical writing and record of your goals. Use it to keep tracking your progress and the barriers and facilitators you can find on the path.

Write it down (Table 8.1): Outline a short description for each detail and follow and enjoy the learning towards your professional and personal progress.

WHAT OUTCOMES?

It is important to set your goals depending on your expectations, especially to understand and learn from those unpredictable situations.

A good first practice when you start chasing your goals practically is to not stick too strongly to them. Try to be flexible and embrace uncertainty, but at the same time rely on the references you are building. Try to make it like the alchemist 'enjoy the journey' and not let it become a cold checklist assessment of the outcomes you achieved.

Keep an eye on and assess your process and where it led you. This leads to a further distinction in GS between process and outcome goals.

Process goals take into consideration actions and aspects that the subject can control and put together to get to the goal. They are related more to what to do and not to the result. They can be useful to build a sense of control over the result and to estimate the difficulties and barriers.

Outcome goals can get out of control (e.g., getting accepted in a ranking for a certain job) and compete not only with our capabilities but also with the capabilities of the people around us.

A second type of categorisation can take into consideration on the time of the terms of the goals. With this in mind, growing awareness of the own level of ability, the importance of creating opportunities and a supporting network can play a huge part in setting realistic aims (Haff & Triplett, 2008).

Short-term goals (e.g., putting into practice your latest reading on the management of patellar tendinopathy) are generally considered a subpart of the overall goal and can help with building an overall goal that makes you feel good, gives you motivation and engages your curiosity.

Medium- and long-term goals (e.g., becoming the number one expert physiotherapist in the world about patellar tendinopathy) can seldom be rewarding, but they work like a frame or a 'target' or destination.

HOW CAN WE MAKE IT HAPPEN?

As mentioned previously, GS should take into consideration factors that can create variability (in terms of barriers or facilitation) around the outcome. Some common practical factors include time, social support, self-awareness, intrinsic motivation in pursuing a goal and the selection and acceptance of a mentor.

This last factor especially could be helpful in identifying a profession and learning what it takes to achieve your short-term and middle-term goals, not only from a career perspective but also from a psychological attitudinal mentorship (Greco & Kraimer, 2020).

Feedback (even an informal moment of self-evaluation or with mentors) can influence and spark emotional reactions, attitudes and behaviours. As in teamwork, focus on positive feedback rather than weighing on negative aspects of your process of professional growth (Salcinovic et al., 2022).

ACHIEVEMENT AND FAILURE

Achievements and eventually failure are not easily defined by some objective criteria due to the highly personal definition of the goal and the unpredictable nature of the extrinsic and intrinsic variables affecting the outcomes.

It would not be surprising that in many situations, achievements can be related to extrinsic factors such as salary, the convenience of a certain job position or, more generally, that some clinicians can be guided by 'self' rather than 'other' (Pearl, 1990).

In clinical and healthcare professions (such as physiotherapy), achievements surely can result strongly from factors such as experience and clinical expertise throughout different areas and infrastructures, roles, responsibility and rewards to be fully appreciated (Rath et al., 2021).

Therefore, it would probably be more appropriate to focus on the acquisition of skills, awareness and self-evaluation of the quality of our own professional growth process.

The definition of success in physiotherapy should take into consideration unpredictable outcomes, such as quality of life and risk of burnout. Therefore, success can be considered highly personal and related to some psychological aspects such as a sense of coherence and coping/adaptive styles in problem-solving. The results probably depend and rely more on personal achievements than academic job-related achievements (Tartas et al., 2011).

GS should not be considered a linear process but a complex system that can evolve together with the person itself, influenced by different aspects of real life and priorities such as family, health, friendships and so on.

It is important to note that a professional should not be ranked or defined by achievement or acquisition, but instead by an internal assessment of how you feel improved and how you contribute to others' growth.

Success has been linked to status or mediated by ego, but we should focus more on the consequences of the trial and the development of the person first, and for the physiotherapist, based on long-term values such as building curiosity, respect of the people around you and integrity.

Not achieving, without any doubt, should be considered in the programming of GS, and not necessarily seen as a failure but a moment of feedback and reflection on the capability to balance expectations and reality and differentiate between the words goal, hope, aspirations and dreams (Soundy et al., 2010).

Create a better awareness of what you were, what you are and what you want to be.

We will now share some interviews with experienced physiotherapists on their career journeys, setting goals and challenges they faced.

Interview 1: Sue Falsone, President and Founder of Structure and Function Education, Director of Movement and Return to Performance for the Houston Texans, Associate Professor of Athletic Training at A. T. Still University

In 2012, at the LA Dodgers, Sue became the first female head athletic trainer to hold that position in any of the four major US sports.

Sue accidentally began a career as a physiotherapist. She had wanted to be an orthopaedic surgeon and had decided to do a physiotherapy degree as her pre-med and fell in love with physiotherapy.

Initially in her career, the opportunities Sue pursued allowed her to build an understanding of what she enjoyed and didn't enjoy.

'There are many standouts in my career, but my ultimate pivotal moment was my very first position in North Carolina in an outpatient orthopaedic clinic. I worked with an athletic trainer there who told me what athletic training was and told me about a program at UNC-Chapel Hill that had a double major in human movement and sports med. Meeting her, and that decision to pursue that graduate education, launched my career in sports medicine, and changed my life in ways I never could have imagined.'

When asked if she set professional goals, she replied,

'I don't. I have never known what I wanted to do. I just always knew what I didn't want to do. And that has been very powerful for me. It has allowed me to consider opportunities I never could have dreamed of.'

Earlier in her career, Sue acknowledged that when she chose opportunities external motivators played a stronger role in her decision making. As her career has progressed and her self-awareness has increased, her decisions have been driven by internal motivators.

'A lot of positions made me choose being a PT OR and AT OR a strength coach. I knew I didn't want to be just one of those. I wanted to be all three. So, I sought positions that allowed me to blend, versus forcing me to pick one.'

Interview 2: Dr Ricky Bell, Māori Physiotherapist and Researcher, Previous Head of the Physiotherapy Program at Waikato Institute of Technology

Ricky also accidentally came to physiotherapy after initially wanting to be a pilot.

Early on in his career, Ricky followed a relatively 'standard' physiotherapy pathway in MSK clinics. With the arrival of his children, he started to question his motivations more deeply, resulting in his family moving to a different country.

It was conversations with his uncle that shifted him towards researching and teaching. The conversations made him aware of his prosocial motivation to impact the health of Māori in New Zealand. He realised that he could create a larger health impact with research that impacted health policy, teaching new physiotherapists about reducing health inequities and creating allyship to promote the health of Māori and Pacific people within the physiotherapy profession in New Zealand.

Ricky acknowledges that at times following this career pathway has been a burden. He has missed out on some family time that he would have enjoyed and has come up against resistance as he has tried to make changes.

Now that Ricky understands his motivations and path, he selects opportunities by asking,

'Is this going to help the pathway for our people on this planet?.'

These days when he sets goals, they are around how he wants to live his life as opposed to outcomes he wants to achieve. He shared goals around wanting to be more connected and present with his loved ones and his environment and his sense of purpose.

'Some physios are doing some cool stuff. And you don't want to reign them in too tight to put the shackles on them so they can't explore those spaces and take our profession as it evolves into what it's going to be tomorrow. That's why we need to listen to our young people more.'

Interview 3: Marco Cuniberti, High-Performance Physiotherapist for Aspire Academy, Doha, Qatar, Lecturer at the University of Siena, Italy, for the MSc in Sports Physiotherapy

Marco's interest in physiotherapy began together with his polyhedric youth sports activity (football, athletics and volleyball), and some injuries occurred. A first aspiration was to improve the quality and standards of care for the people facing the same issues and provide better knowledge and understanding.

'Like many other professionals, I have gained experience in my own cabinet with amateur sportsmen where I had the opportunity to get out of my comfort zone and face the importance of new responsibilities and boosted my management and rehabilitation skills after my MSc in sports physiotherapy, where I had the opportunity to start collaborations with national teams and elite athletes.'

Marco had the chance to move to Doha in 2017, attracted by the potentiality of a high-profile job perspective, increasing his responsibilities and salary perspectives. Also he found particularly appealing the opportunity to cope with a new culture, in a new country (from Italy to Qatar) and working with world-class physiotherapists and other colleagues.

'This kind of experience definitely led me to have a better perspective of my own goals. I developed a sense of acceptance about the adjustable and modifiable nature of this process since I've started to learn that a lot of things can change in the short and midterm. It can even be totally different from what you set at the beginning of the career. It takes time before you can clearly have awareness.'

The overall considerations about his journey are positive anyway: he daily deals with different mindsets, genders, religions and experiences and has had the opportunity to have realistic expectations in terms of fixing achievable objectives with the same curiosity and ambition.

His view of a successful mindset is defined by the achievement of patient-related professional outcomes and a subjective feeling of 'Get home, sleep with calm and peacefulness and start the day with enthusiasm to face the new challenges of the day'.

Five Key Takeaways

1. Start with the end in mind. Give yourself a long-term goal and try to understand what it takes to reach it. Then try to self-assess your needs in terms of education and hard and soft skills. Plan a strategy to integrate them into your personal and professional process of growth.
2. The process of GS is highly subjective and should take into consideration and balance personal beliefs, passions and necessity. It should involve the people around you and possibly follow a SMART(ER) approach.
3. The destination or direction and the terms can be fixed, but with the same awareness of the high degree of variables that can make them change or be redefined.
4. Despite the huge number of possibilities, define what is meaningful for you, try to accept the uncertainty and, once you decide on your path, go for it. Try not to be frustrated by other possibilities and alternatives.
5. Focus on the process of learning and skills acquisition, and with serendipity give yourself a moment of self-evaluation based on appreciating what you learned, and, if needed, give your professional priorities a new direction.

Five Self-Directed Reflections

1. What are the process and outcome goals in your own professional journey, and how do you balance between them in your overall goal-setting strategy?
2. How have your short-term and long-term goals evolved over time, and how does this evolution reflect your personal growth and changing circumstances?
3. How do you identify and overcome barriers that might hinder your progress towards achieving your goals? What role does mentorship and feedback play in this process?
4. How do you define success and failure in your professional journey, and how does this definition shape your self-perception and motivation?
5. Reflecting on the interviews provided, what resonates with you the most from everyone's journey, and how can you incorporate these insights into your own professional development and goal-setting strategy?

References

Reid, A., & Dixon, H. (2018). Making sense of the numbers: Analysis of the physiotherapy workforce. *Berl,* 1–36. Available at https://pnz.org.nz/Folder?Action=View%20File&Folder_id=1&File=PNZ%20Workforce%20Issues%20December%202018.pdf. Accessed 15 March 2024.

Bulley, C., Donaghy, M., Coppoolse, R., Bizzini, M., van Cingel, R., DeCarlo, M., Dekker, L., Grant, M., Meeusen, R., Phillips, N., & Risberg, M. (2004). Sports Physiotherapy Competencies and Standards. *Sports Physiotherapy for All Project.*

Carmona-Barrientos, I., Gala-León, F. J., & Lupiani-Giménez, M. (2020). Occupational stress and burnout among physiotherapists: A cross-sectional survey in Cadiz (Spain). *Human Resources for Health, 18,* 91. https://doi.org/10.1186/s12960-020-00537-0.

Carse, J. (2011). *Finite and infinite games.* New York, NY: Simon and Schuster.

Chia, L., Taylor, D., Pappas, E., Hegedus, E. J., & Michener, L. A. (2022). Beginning with the end in mind: Implementing backward design to improve sports injury rehabilitation practices. *Journal of Orthopedic Sports Physical Therapy, 52*(12), 770–776. https://doi.org/10.2519/jospt.2022.11440.

Coppack, R. J., Kristensen, J., & Karageorghis, C. I. (2012). Use of a goal setting intervention to increase adherence to low back pain rehabilitation: A randomised controlled trial. *Clinical Rehabilitation, 26,* 1032–1042.

Covey, S. R., & Covey, S. (2020). *The 7 habits of highly effective people.* New York, NY: Simon & Schuster.

Deci, E. L., & Ryan, R. M. (1991). A motivational approach to self: Integration in personality. In Dienstbier, R. A. (Ed.), *Nebraska Symposium on Motivation, 1990: Perspectives on motivation* (pp. 237–288). Lincon, NE: University of Nebraska Press.

Deci, E. L., & Ryan, R. M. (1995). *Human autonomy.* In M. H. Kernis (Ed.), *Efficacy, agency, and self-esteem* (pp. 31–49). Boston, MA: Springer.

Dekker, J., de Groot, V., Ter Steeg, A. M., Vloothuis, J., Holla, J., Collette, E., … Littooij, E. (2020). Setting meaningful goals in rehabilitation: Rationale and practical tools. *Clinical Rehabilitation, 34*(1), 3–12. https://doi.org/10.1177/0269215519876299.

González-Sánchez, B., López-Arza, M. V. G., Montanero-Fernández, J., Varela-Donoso, E., Rodríguez-Mansilla, J., & Mingote-Adán, J. C. (2017). Burnout syndrome prevalence in physiotherapists. *Revista da Associação Médica Brasileira, 63,* 361–365.

Grant, A. M. (2008). Does intrinsic motivation fuel the prosocial fire? Motivational synergy in predicting persistence, performance, and productivity. *Journal of Applied Psychology, 93*(1), 48.

Grant, A. M., & Berg, J. M (2012). Prosocial motivation. In Cameron, K. S., & Spreitzer, G. M. (Eds.), *The Oxford handbook of positive organizational scholarship* (pp. 28–44). New York, NY: Oxford University Press.

Grant, A. M., & Berry, J. W. (2011). The necessity of others is the mother of invention: Intrinsic and prosocial motivations, perspective taking, and creativity. *Academy of Management Journal, 54*(1), 73–96.

Greco, L. M., & Kraimer, M. L. (2020). Goal setting in the career management process: An identity theory perspective. *Journal of Applied Psychology, 105*(1), 40–57.

Haff, G., & Triplett, N. (2008). *Essentials of strength training and conditioning. National Strength and Conditioning Association* (pp. 168–169). Champaign, IL: Human Kinetics, 2016

Hammond, R., Cross, V., & Moore, A. (2016). The construction of professional identity by physiotherapists: A qualitative study. *Physiotherapy, 102*(1), 71–77. https://doi.org/10.1016/j.physio.2015.04.002.

Latzke, M., Putz, P., Kulnik, S. T., Schlegl, C., Sorge, M., & Mériaux-Kratochvila, S. (2021). Physiotherapists' job satisfaction according to employment situation: Findings from an online survey in Austria. *Physiotherapy Research International, 26*(3), e1907.

Mazerolle, S. M., Eason, C. M., Ferraro, E. M., & Goodman, A. (2015). Career and family aspirations of female athletic trainers employed in the National Collegiate Athletic Association Division I setting. *Journal of Athletic Training, 50*(2), 170–177. https://doi.org/10.4085/1062-6050-49.3.59.

Nix, G. A., Ryan, R. M., Manly, J. B., & Deci, E. L. (1999). Revitalization through self-regulation: The effects of autonomous and controlled motivation on happiness and vitality. *Journal of Experimental Social Psychology, 35*(3), 266–284.

Øster, I., Munk, K., & Henriksen, J. (2017). Career dreams among health care students: I want to make a difference. *Gerontology & Geriatrics Education*, 1–14. https://doi.org/10.1080/02701960.2017.1311881.

Pearl, M. J. (1990). Factors physical therapists use to make career decisions. *Physical Therapy, 70*(2), 105–107. https://doi.org/10.1093/ptj/70.2.105.

Rath, L., Faletra, A., Downing, N., & Rushton, A. (2021). Cross-sectional survey of advanced practice physiotherapy: Characteristics and perceptions of existing roles. *International Journal of Therapy and Rehabilitation*. https://doi.org/10.12968/ijtr.2020.0064.

Rose, T., & Ogas, O. (2018). *Dark horse: Achieving success through the pursuit of fulfillment.* New York, NY: HarperCollins.

Rose, L. T., Rouhani, P., & Fischer, K. W. (2013). The science of the individual. *Mind, Brain, and Education, 7*(3), 152–158.

Ryan, R. M. (1995). Psychological needs and the facilitation of integrative processes. *Journal of Personality, 63*(3), 397–427.

Ryan, R. M., & Deci, E. L. (2000). Intrinsic and extrinsic motivations: Classic definitions and new directions. *Contemporary Educational Psychology, 25*(1), 54–67. https://doi.org/10.1006/ceps.1999.1020.

Ryan, R. M., Deci, E. L., & Grolnick, W. S. (1995). Autonomy, relatedness, and the self: Their relation to development and psychopathology. In Cicchetti, D., & Cohen, D. J. (Eds.), *Developmental psychopathology*, Vol. 1. Theory and methods (pp. 618–655). Hoboken, NJ: John Wiley & Sons.

Salcinovic, B., Drew, M., & Dijkstra, P. (2022). Factors influencing team performance: What can support teams in high-performance sport learn from other industries? A systematic scoping review. *Sports Medicine – Open, 8*, 25. https://doi.org/10.1186/s40798-021-00406-7.

Scobbie, L., Dixon, D., & Wyke, S. (2011). Goal setting and action planning in the rehabilitation setting: Development of a theoretically informed practice framework. *Clinical Rehabilitation, 25*(5), 468–482. https://doi.org/10.1177/0269215510389198.

Sheldon, K. M., Ryan, R. M., Rawsthorne, L. J., & Ilardi, B. (1997). Trait self and true self: Cross-role variation in the Big-Five personality traits and its relations with psychological authenticity and subjective well-being. *Journal of Personality and Social Psychology, 73*(6), 1380.

Soundy, A., Smith, B., Butler, M., Minns Lowe, C., Helen, D., & Winward, C. H. (2010). A qualitative study in neurological physiotherapy and hope: Beyond physical improvement. *Physiotherapy Theory and Practice, 26*(2), 79–88. https://doi.org/10.3109/09593980802634466.

Stevens, A., Köke, A., van der Weijden, T., & Beurskens, A. (2017). Ready for goal setting? Process evaluation of a patient-specific goal-setting method in physiotherapy. *BMC Health Services Research, 17*(1), 618. https://doi.org/10.1186/s12913-017-2557-9.

Tartas, M., Walkiewicz, M., Majkowicz, M., & Budzinski, W. (2011). Psychological factors determining success in a medical career: A 10-year longitudinal study. *Medical Teacher, 33*(3), e163–e172. https://doi.org/10.3109/0142159X.2011.54479.

Tian, X., Peng, X., & Peng, X. (2021). Influence of prosocial motivation on employee creativity: The moderating role of regulatory focus and the mediating role of knowledge sharing. *Frontiers in Psychology 12*, 3880.

University of California. (2017). *Smart goals, a how to guide, performance appraisal planning 2016–2017.* Available at https://www.ucop.edu/local-human-resources/_files/performanceappraisal/How%20to%20write%20SMART%20Goals%20v2.pdf.

Wade, D. T. (2009). Goal setting in rehabilitation: An overview of what, why and how. *Clinical Rehabilitation, 23*(4), 291–295.

World Physiotherapy Association. (n.d.). Advocacy/rehabilitation. Available at https://world.physio/advocacy/rehabilitation. Accessed 4 March 2024.

CHAPTER 9

Personal Brand Design

Steph Allen

> *'It's easier to change yourself than to change the world. And the best way to change the world is to change yourself.'*
> – Naval Ravikant, entrepreneur, investor and cofounder of AngelList, in *Almanack of Naval Ravikant* by Eric Jorgenson, 2020

CHAPTER OUTLINE

Introduction
How Did I Get Here?
The Influence and Guidance of Mentors
Taking the Leap, Leading With Your Why and Shaping Your Brand

Build Your Business Around Your Life, Not Your Life Around Your Business
Challenges
Bringing It All Together
Five Key Takeaways
Five Self-Directed Reflections

Introduction

I am going to begin this chapter with a confession: I once had a lot of negative feelings towards physio/physical therapists who were 'promoting their brand'. I associated this self-promotion with financial interests rather than caring about patients or clients. Granted, there were and will always be some individuals out there who have less than genuine intentions; we should not make sweeping declarations or generalisations. It wasn't until I started to feel frustrated in my clinical role that I even had the smallest thought of creating my own thing. I knew that my intentions were genuine, so then perhaps my judgement of others creating their own thing was a bit harsh. And so I decided to question my previous judgement of that dirty word 'brand'.

How Did I Get Here?

Allow me to provide some context with a piece of my story: my 'how did I get here?' journey. As a new graduate physical therapist (PT), I was utterly terrified of having full autonomy over a caseload of patients. Even after completing a yearlong orthopaedic residency and receiving my orthopaedic certified specialist (OCS) designation, there was that lingering imposter syndrome. I opted to pursue travel physical therapy, and it was here that a fire started to burn within me.

I'd had an underlying interest in anterior cruciate ligament (ACL) rehabilitation since my own ACL injury in high school. During travel PT, however, I realised that the quality of ACL rehab left a lot to be desired, especially for the high-level athlete/individual. Sadly, it didn't seem to change much across state lines in the United States where I work. I turned to the literature for some solace, only to find out that the numbers gathered there seemed to echo what I was seeing in terms of poor long-term outcomes, high retear rates and minimal consistency in return to sport testing (if any formal testing was done at all) (Joreitz *et al.*, 2016, Toole *et al.*, 2017, Cristiani *et al.*, 2019). This frustration would later serve as my primary 'why' and would ultimately lead to me connecting with like-minded individuals who have now become my most trusted and respected mentors and friends.

After about 2 years doing travel PT, I had gained some clinical confidence and was ready to continue to hone my skills and primarily serve the ACL population. I landed a full-time position at an amazing sports-focused clinic in the Boston area, and I was finally living out what I dreamed of during my time travelling. That was until the majority of my caseload became filled working with those who were going through ACL rehabilitation. I ran into more roadblocks. First, insurance in the United States often cuts people off long before they are ready to fully return to their sport or activity. Second, for most patients in the insurance model, I was only able to see people 2 (or maybe 3) days per week, with little oversight as to what they were doing for the other 4 to 5 days of the week. I realised quickly that most individuals were not consistent in between sessions. This does not prepare a person well for a successful return to sport or high-level activity. But what could I do? I only had control over what they were doing for 40 to 60 minutes with me in the clinic twice a week and had little to no influence on what they did outside of those times.

My solution included the following: programming for all of my patients for their out-of-clinic days so that we could spread out their limited number of visits, spending a ridiculous amount of time on the phone with insurance companies and writing progress notes every other week in order to try to get more visits approved. This worked . . . for a while. It worked until I completely burnt out because 40 hours of clinical care turned into likely 60 hours, a good bit of which I was not being compensated for.

All I kept thinking was, 'There has to be a better way to serve the ACL population without the clinician sacrificing their quality of life!' I hadn't the slightest idea what I could do about this, so I did what I usually do when I felt stuck clinically: I looked at those who I respect and who were already doing what I wanted to potentially do, and I reached out to my mentors.

The Influence and Guidance of Mentors

KEY POINT 1: YOU NEVER KNOW HOW AUTHENTIC CONNECTIONS MAY INFLUENCE YOU AND SERVE YOUR MISSION

I would like to acknowledge those who made me believe that it was even possible to start something of my own for 'ACL-ers'. I also hope that sharing how this all organically unfolded will reassure students and young clinicians that finding mentors doesn't always have to be overly formal or strategic.

In 2018, my partner and I cofounded an education/mentorship company called The Level Up Initiative. The idea to move forward and create this company was entirely his, as I was still not at a point where I was confident enough to make that type of leap. However, I was in full support because it was fuelled by such a strong mission, born out of our frustrations surrounding the harmful misinformation that was affecting our patients.

Our mission for The Level Up Initiative is to 'transform the people that will transform healthcare'. My partner and I merged The Level Up Initiative with a like-minded company, Clinical Athlete, in 2021, and became Clinical Athlete & Level Up (CALU). Our collective mission and reach are growing by the day. Being a part of this group and seeing that it is possible to take an idea and create something from it planted the seed for me. It allowed me to see that all of us at CALU could start at ground zero and build something of meaning and influence and that as PTs we can do more than just treat clients in the clinic.

Between 2018 and now, I began to interact more with individuals on social media that seemed to share my frustrations and motivations around the same things in the ACL rehab realm. Connecting with people, asking conceptual-based questions and even commiserating on different topics led to the relationships that now are so important to me and help push me to learn more and continue to be a better clinician and coach to this day. Interacting authentically with others, asking questions and being open to being wrong are ways that I developed my 'challenge network', as Adam Grant calls it (Grant, 2021). It really does come down to entering conversations and relationships with genuine curiosity rather than simply trying to fulfil expectations.

The final piece to it all was more formal coaching and guidance in the process of creating my business because, let's be real, most PTs are not well versed in the business side of things. For this, I am ever thankful to have found and joined the Honey Badger Project, an incubator for mission-driven businesses. Their mission and values are very well aligned with both my own and ours at CALU, and I truly believe that what they are doing is going to help change healthcare at large.

I feel incredibly fortunate to have the people behind me that I do, and I am here to reassure you that it is not all about luck. It requires putting yourself out there, being vulnerable and forging meaningful relationships with others.

Once I felt like I had my squad behind me, I was ready to take the leap, as ready as I'd ever feel. This brings up another important point, however. I believe that you cannot take a confident initial leap without a strong 'why'. So, let's talk about that!

Taking the Leap, Leading With Your Why and Shaping Your Brand

I mentioned earlier that my frustration with the standard of care for those who have suffered an ACL injury would serve as the kindling for my fire. This remains true to this day – the kindling is plentiful. Here is why: I see myself in so many of my patients and clients. So many people do not receive the support and guidance they need in their ACL rehab process and the consequences are life altering. That is not an exaggeration. My life was altered in a negative way by the lack of guidance and education I received in my rehab journey, and I will die trying to make sure that that doesn't happen for others – because it doesn't have to! We have the knowledge and tools to mitigate future risk and improve quality of life after this injury and we simply do not do a good job of utilising the knowledge in our guidance of people through this process.

This is what I believe it requires to develop your mission and core values, and take your first leap in creating your brand and your impact. Your mission and values, fuelled by your 'why', are essentially your launch pad.

KEY POINT 2: MISSION/CORE VALUES + A STRONG WHY + GENUINE CONNECTIONS = POWERFUL LAUNCH PAD FOR YOUR PERSONAL BRAND

'Authenticity means erasing the gap between what you firmly believe inside and what you reveal to the outside world.'

> – ADAM GRANT, PROFESSOR AT THE WHARTON
> SCHOOL OF THE UNIVERSITY OF PENNSYLVANIA

My mission started with *who* I wanted to reach. From day one, I had a very clear picture of the ideal clients whom I would serve and guide.

I launched ACLResolve with the mission to create a space for 'ACL-ers', devoid of outside noise, where they can redefine their identity and begin their journey to becoming the strongest mental and physical versions of themselves. This mission is fuelled by core values of humility, integrity, empathy, passion and fun. This is what comes through in my branding and messaging.

I also believe it is vital to be the same person on social media that you are in your day-to-day life. This will be something that I will always strive for, even as ACLResolve grows and evolves.

Operating from this place as your authentic self, motivated by this mission, you cannot fail. You can only make mistakes, learn from them and keep moving forward. Speaking of moving forward, though, you'll need a road map to move at all. That is where a business model comes in.

I had never thought about creating a business model. I had just gotten past internal resistance to even believe that I could do this! This is not a chapter on the logistics of business model building, but it is worth mentioning that this is important and that it should be built around your ideal life design, not the other way around.

I think that many of us who have such passion in an area get ahead of ourselves and just throw ourselves into the business, trading one form of burnout for another. That will be the fastest way to put out your fire and make you forget why you started all of this in the first place. So listen up because this is the best advice I've ever received.

Build Your Business Around Your Life, Not Your Life Around Your Business

I tell myself this all the time.

With that being said, you do also need to put some pieces in place to create your minimum viable product (MVP). For ACLResolve, for example, I needed to decide if I was going to be having people enrol on a month-to-month basis or ask that they commit to a longer time frame initially. I also needed to decide what would be an ethical and sustainable starting rate for services. A lot of these questions arose, and it took time to answer them, but these are the types of questions you need to be asking yourself during the creation process.

Then, with each iteration of your MVP, you must ask yourself, 'Does this model serve the individuals I am trying to reach?' This is why it is so important to have a clearly defined picture of these individuals. Now, in all of your messaging, you are talking directly to them, and that can be an incredibly powerful means of lead generation for your business. Imagine how amazing it would feel to know that what you are putting out into the world as your true, authentic self is reaching exactly who you want to work with and making them feel heard!

KEY POINT 3: EVERYTHING WILL CHANGE AND EVOLVE

Do not let that stall you in making these initial decisions. I think of it like strength testing in ACL rehab: these numbers are information only. They do not dictate what type of person the athlete is. They just tell us where we need to go next.

People, society, trends and data – these will all change. Allow yourself and your business to change as well. Consider this: If we don't change and grow as time goes on, are we truly remaining authentic anyway?

KEY POINT 4: IN TAKING YOUR LEAP AND GROWING YOUR BRAND, BUSINESS AND IMPACT, YOU MUST CONTINUALLY TAKE UNCERTAIN ACTION

Knowing that things will continue to evolve, you can ensure that they evolve in a net positive direction if you are always taking action. Even when you are doing something for the first time and are not sure what the outcome will be, you won't know for sure unless you try. Obviously, you want to make informed decisions so that you are taking calculated risks versus blind risks, but you still want to act.

Then, you adapt and evolve based on what you learn from each action (every action has a reaction, right?). This simple concept has allowed me to grow and learn so much, and even though not everything I've tried has worked, I am still in business and growing and learning. I'll take that!

Challenges

Your personal brand and anything born from it will be challenged at times. Therefore, you will feel resistance, struggle and uncertainty. However, I prefer to view challenge in a positive, motivating light whenever I can (confession: it is not easy). The definition of challenge, as a noun, in the Merriam-Webster dictionary is as follows: A stimulating task or problem (Merriam-Webster, n.d.). That doesn't sound so anxiety provoking when we think of it that way, right?

I have experienced difficulties thus far in building something from my personal brand, and I expect to face plenty more in the future as I learn and grow. For starters, I had immense imposter syndrome (see Fig. 9.1). I still experience it from time to time but have worked hard to keep it in check. For those unfamiliar with this term, imposter syndrome is a psychological condition that is characterised by persistent doubt concerning one's abilities or accomplishments, accompanied by the fear of being exposed as a fraud despite evidence of one's ongoing success (Merriam-Webster, n.d.). The problem with imposter syndrome is that it can result in procrastination, overpreparation, attributing your successes to things other than yourself and ultimately a lot of anxiety and/or depression (Feigofsky, 2022).

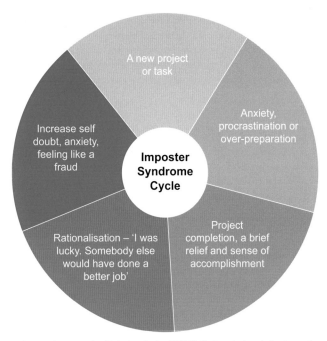

Fig. 9.1   The imposter syndrome cycle. (Data Incubator. [2022]. *6 steps to break the imposter syndrome cycle.* https://www.thedataincubator.com/blog/2022/02/23/6-steps-to-break-the-imposter-syndrome-cycle/.)

The dialogue in my own head sounded like this: 'Am I smart and capable enough to do this? Are people going to find out that I don't know everything? Am I crazy to think I can start something while also still working in the clinic?' I had a pretty steady stream of this questioning early on, which was clearly not conducive to learning and growing. This was quite a stimulating problem that I needed to figure out. Although it comes in waves, still, I have been able to work through this and create mental space to push forward.

I also felt some internal resistance as I began to manage a small team of people within ACLResolve. I had never been in that type of position before, and the task for me was to figure out how to remain in a place of leadership but also work with others as equals and team members. Making sure that the ecosystem I create remains safe, collaborative and productive has always been important to me, but this too is something that needs to be figured out. It's a challenge in and of itself.

Perhaps the biggest challenge I still have is ensuring that I do not trade one form of burnout for another. Part of the reason I even took this leap is that I couldn't give my best in the clinic anymore. It had gotten to be too much, and I felt my passion being smothered. I am not sure what true success looks like, but I know that it does NOT involve burning out on your own accord. This is likely something that a lot of entrepreneurs go through, and so I feel it is worth touching on here. Passion and a strong mission can motivate you to do so much early on, but keeping guardrails up is important so you don't run yourself off the road to fulfilling your mission.

Bringing It All Together

In full transparency, I was not consciously working to build a brand through this journey. Hindsight has allowed me to see that I was doing just that all along. That has led me to reflect and share these experiences with you in the hope that it can help you in building your authentic brand if that is what you aim to do. So, let's bring it all together!

To create your personal brand, and to build anything from it, requires you to set yourself apart from others in a positive manner. It needs to be fuelled by passion and an unwavering mission. It is an ongoing process, throughout which you are promoting yourself and trying new things, and then reflecting, learning and adjusting as you move forward. Here are some of the key steps involved in building a personal brand for a physiotherapist, from my experience:

Five Key Takeaways

1. Define your niche and develop your brand identity: Determine the area of expertise or interest that you want to build your brand around. What fires you up and inspires you to want to serve a particular population? Create a brand identity that reflects your mission and values, personality and skills. This could include a logo, website, social media presence, brand voice and other marketing materials.
2. Establish your online presence: Create social media profiles and potentially a website to showcase your skills and achievements, as well as the mission and intent of your brand. Engage with your followers, create content and share your expertise.
3. Network and build relationships: Attend conferences and seminars, join professional organisations and connect with like-minded individuals to build a network of contacts. These connections can help you gain visibility and credibility.
4. Be authentic and consistent and keep developing your skills: Your personal brand should reflect who you are, your values and your goals. Everyone who comes in contact with your brand should know why it was started in the first place. Be consistent in your messaging and ensure that your actions align with your brand. Be the same person on social media you are in your day-to-day life. Keep learning in your field to enhance your expertise and

reputation. This could include attending conferences, taking courses or participating in online training programs. It also includes continually asking questions both of ourselves and of what we have learned to foster solid critical thinking and clinical judgement.

5. Continually monitor and adjust: Keep track of how your personal brand is perceived and adjust your strategy accordingly. Continuously assess and refine your brand presence to ensure that it reflects your evolving goals and aspirations. People grow and evolve – allow your brand to do the same, and people will appreciate that.

Five Self-Directed Reflections

1. The relentless pull I have always had towards improving the standard for ACL rehab has been a guiding light for me in my journey. What's your guiding light?
2. I was not deliberately building a brand for much of my journey, which led to the emphasis on building genuine relationships with mentors and colleagues. This was my springboard. Map out your relationships.
3. Imposter syndrome does not fully go away for me, but continually taking action in different facets of my business helps it influence me less and less. Do you feel like an imposter sometimes? What do you do about it?
4. Committing to this process of creating a business and brand and fulfilling my mission continues to be one of the greatest influences on my own confidence. Can you commit to building something for you?
5. The ups and downs of an entrepreneurial path have taught me to be humble and persistent, the combination of which I believe can foster great accomplishments. Can you adopt a mindset like this even if you don't run your own business?

References

Cristiani, R., Mikkelsen, C., Forssblad, M., Engström, B., & Stålman, A. (2019). Only one patient out of five achieves symmetrical knee function 6 months after primary anterior cruciate ligament reconstruction. *Knee Surgery, Sports Traumatology, Arthroscopy, 27*(11), 3461–3470. https://doi.org/10.1007/s00167-019-05396-4.

Feigofsky, S. (2022). Imposter syndrome. *Heart Rhythm Case Reports, 8*(12), 861–862. https://doi.org/10.1016/j.hrcr.2022.11.001.

Grant, A. (2021). *Think Again: The Power of Knowing What You Don't Know*. Viking/Penguin Random House.

Joreitz, R., Lynch, A., Rabuck, S., Lynch, B., Davin, S., & Irrgang, J. (2016). Patient-specific and surgery-specific factors that affect return to sport after ACL reconstruction. *International Journal of Sports Physical Therapy, 11*(2), 264–278.

Jorgenson, E. (2020). *The almanack of Naval Ravikant: A guide to wealth and happiness*. Magrathea Publishing.

Merriam-Webster. (n.d.). *Challenge*. In Merriam-Webster.com Dictionary. Available at https://www.merriam-webster.com/dictionary/challenge. Accessed 25 April 2023.

Merriam-Webster. (n.d.). *Impostor syndrome*. In Merriam-Webster.com Dictionary. Available at https://www.merriam-webster.com/dictionary/impostor%20syndrome. Accessed 25 April 2023.

The Data Incubator. (2022). *6 steps to break the imposter syndrome cycle*. Available at https://www.thedataincubator.com/blog/2022/02/23/6-steps-to-break-the-imposter-syndrome-cycle/. Accessed 20 January 2024.

Toole, A., Ithurburn, M., Rauh, M., Hewett, T., Paterno, M., & Schmitt, L. (2017). Young athletes cleared for sports participation after anterior cruciate ligament reconstruction: How many actually meet recommended return-to-sport criterion cutoffs? *Journal of Orthopaedic & Sports Physical Therapy, 47*(11), 825–833. https://doi.org/10.2519/jospt.2017.7227.

Performance

CHAPTER 10

Mental Fitness – Resilience and Facing Challenges

Darren Finnegan ▪ Chrystal Lynch

'If I were a Dr., I'd prescribe books. They can be just as powerful as drugs.'
– Shane Parrish, founder, curator, and wisdom seeker behind Farnam Street and author of
The Great Mental Models

Introduction

Mental fitness has a different meaning for many people. I am sure you will have worked with individuals who are physically conditioned, are emotionally intelligent and possess an optimistic mindset. However, what happens when they face a situation outside of their control, a setback or an adverse life situation?

This is where the components of 'resilience' become important.

Martin Seligman is known as the godfather of positive psychology. He has done extensive research into helplessness, optimism, happiness and wellbeing (Seligman, 2011). He was responsible for developing the Penn Resilience Program (PRP) used within the military and several other sectors. They started the program by exploring military personnel's understanding of post-traumatic stress disorder (PTSD; of which 97% of them were familiar with the term). However, only 10% of the soldiers interviewed had ever heard of 'post-traumatic growth' (Seligman *et al.*, 2018).

If we are only aware of the negative construct (in this case, PTSD), this will be how we view the world in challenging times. This may then lead to rumination, fear, avoidance and catastrophising, which is the greatest risk factor for those developing chronic musculoskeletal problems (Petrini & Arendt-Nielsen, 2020).

Have you ever stopped to think about what the positive components of psychology are?

We all have mental health – the thoughts, beliefs and experiences that have shaped how we view the world on a cognitive level. It is estimated that ill mental health costs the healthcare services £70–100 billion per year in the United Kingdom (Henderson *et al.*, 2014).

If the context within which the world views mental health is only negative, society requires a reframing to understand the positive aspects of our mental health and wellbeing.

Seligman has investigated this extensively, creating a framework based on four domains:

- Physical
- Emotional
- Mental
- Spiritual

The core underpinnings of these domains relate to:

- **Challenges:** the ability to reframe a setback into an opportunity to learn, grow and find solutions.
- **Control:** understanding the autonomy we have in our life, focusing on controllable factors and accepting those outside of our individual control.
- **Commitment:** defining a just cause, purpose or meaning worthy enough to dedicate your life towards.

There will be lessons to learn along the way that may force you to explore your own relationship with facing challenges. This will develop your own inner resilience and enhance your mental fitness for a career in healthcare.

This chapter will intertwine my own past experiences, practical application and lessons for clinical practice through the medium of stories to enhance your reading journey.

Self Awareness

PART 1: FROM PAIN COMES PROGRESS

'He who knows his why, can endure any how.'
    – FRIEDRICH NIETZSCHE, PHILOSOPHER, PROSE POET, CULTURAL CRITIC AND PHILOLOGIST

In my teenage years, I realised the difficulties that my parents faced whilst running a business, a farm and raising a family. This was compounded by my father's alcohol dependency. My dad was a heavy smoker, a workaholic and a poor sleeper, and he survived on a diet that consisted solely of T-bone steaks, two fried eggs and white bread for each meal. I never saw him eat a single vegetable, have a glass of water or do any non-work-related physical activity.

Looking back on it now, it is unsurprising I developed a passion for public health, with a keen interest in addressing modifiable lifestyle factors and rehabilitation.

After several years of fighting against the ill effects of his lifestyle choices, my dad sustained several heart attacks and strokes and, sadly, died when I was 18 years old. This proved a defining point in my life: to decide which path I wanted to follow.

I chose a life of exercise and learning. Immediately following his death, I became relentless in studying for my final exams, only taking breaks to go for runs and to eat.

I had attended physio appointments with dad following his stroke and thought I could help with his rehabilitation. I chose a life of helping others as I felt I had failed to help my dad overcome his biggest challenge.

I chose a life of service to others. I chose a career in physiotherapy. I did not waiver in my decision to study physiotherapy and only became more determined by the day. Motivation for any pursuit is temporary; it will wax and wane over time, but to this day, I have never doubted that I am living my purpose.

If you can find a deeper purpose … it will be an eternal energetic flame providing a relentless drive to keep you moving forward and help you to overcome even the most seemingly insurmountable obstacles. Know your why!

APPLICATION TO CLINICAL PRACTICE

As healthcare professionals, the will to help others can come at the cost of our own wellbeing at times. This may involve doing overtime, a crisis of confidence, staying late at work researching

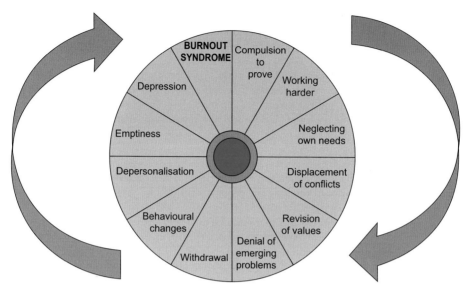

Fig. 10.1 Burnout syndrome. (Adapted with permission from Freudenberger, H. J. [1982]. Counseling and dynamics: treating the end-stage person. In J. W. Jones (Ed.), *The burnout syndrome*. Park Ridge, IL: London House Press; Sirois, F., Owens, J., & Hirsch, J. [2020]. Burnout in healthcare workers: prevalence, impact and preventative strategies. *Local and Regional Anesthesia, 13*, 171–183. https://doi.org/10.2147/LRA.S240564.)

the latest peer-reviewed article and so forth. Burnout in healthcare manifests when we become disconnected from the duty to serve others (De Hert, 2020).

At all stages of your career, it is recommended to improve your self-awareness, an ability to pay attention to thoughts, emotions and responses – and to set professional boundaries to ensure that relentless drive from a defined purpose does not culminate in burnout (Fig. 10.1).

Self-awareness provides a launchpad to understand the 'why' you do what you do and the insight to leverage it for your career to take off. Do not let it be a burden to your own wellbeing. Your career is a marathon, not a sprint. Plan accordingly.

Physical Domain

PART 2: WHAT ARE YOU UNWILLING TO FEEL OR EXPERIENCE?

The choice was made. The decision to commit to working in healthcare. Trusting in the process to get there helped reframe my suffering into helping others.

I decided to push myself in the fields of physiotherapy and fitness – exploring everything about health and wellbeing with an insatiable curiosity. I practised what I preached … pushing myself in physical and academic pursuits to escape the emotion and reality of my situation. My own existential crisis through grief!

The notion of bereavement counselling was absurd to say the least in rural Ireland, especially in my somewhat emotionally stunted family.

My route into physio began at Carlow's Institute of Technology studying Physiology and Health Science. I recall being out for a run on a torrentially wet Irish autumn evening. The world was closing in on me. This vivid memory evokes a world of pain, even to this day, 17 years later.

I had displayed ninja-like skills in concealing any remnants of emotion, deflecting with humour. I had perfected burying any sign of sadness, grief or shame under a façade of partying, alcohol, drugs and exercise.

This night was different.

I ran as fast as I possibly could, hoping if I pushed myself to the point of physical exhaustion, it would again curtail these pesky emotions. I quickly realised this helped to distract from the overwhelming thoughts of my dad. I would get into my body and push as hard and fast as I could. I had accidentally discovered a coping mechanism that appeared to serve me well at the time.

THE BREAK POINT

I pushed myself through a 10-km route at a blistering pace to physical and emotional exhaustion. I stood roadside simultaneously vomiting and crying uncontrollably – a feat that I could not even fathom as humanly possible today.

I came out of my trance for a second to realise a car pulling in beside me. An elderly lady kindly gestured to see if I was OK. She empathetically offered to drive me home to get out of the rain. At this point, the tears blended in with the ice-cold raindrops trickling down my cheeks. I smiled at her warm, welcoming, waving hand. The feeling of shame, guilt and sadness dissipated within me for a minute at her kind gesture. I gratefully refused the offer to avoid the awkward conversation in the car.

She remarked as she drove away, 'My son does the same; young men and their emotions!' I wonder if she realised quite how perceptive she had been!

I stood roadside beside a messy tsunami of vomit at my feet coupled with bright red, puffy eyes. I was trying to piece together her closing comment. I walked home dumbfounded, scratching my head in the rain.

At that precise moment, I would have rather cut off my arm than explore the emotions that were bubbling beneath the surface of my consciousness.

APPLICATION TO CLINICAL PRACTICE

A key resilience competency is self-regulation. This refers to the manner in which you can change your thoughts, behaviours or physiology for a desired outcome (Pincus *et al.*, 2013).

'Between a stimulus and a response, there is a space. In that space, lies the power to choose your response. In our response lies our growth and freedom.'
– VIKTOR FRANKL, AUSTRIAN PSYCHOLOGIST, AUTHOR AND
CONCENTRATION CAMP SURVIVOR

In this example, running was the tool used to deal with the thoughts, changing my physiology and avoiding the emotional turmoil of grief. There is a lot of research on the benefits of any exercise, especially for those with mood disorders, depression and anxiety (Kandola, 2020). All consultations must ensure we help patients break down barriers to engaging in physical activity, for those who are inactive (Pelletier *et al.*, 2017).

We also need to be mindful of when exercise is not the answer to a person's problem; hence addressing the emotional, mental or spiritual domain is indicated. The promotion of talking therapies, social connection, gratitude journaling and meditative practices could be encouraged to help a person deal with the uncomfortable sensation arising and help calm an unsettled mind in the clinic.

Metacognition and self-regulatory skills are developed during childhood through the medium of play (Whitebread *et al.*, 2009). Exercise prescription can be a creative process, filled with innovation and playfulness. It is where the artistic nature of a therapist is tested, to create a therapeutic alliance dance enhancing a patient's self-regulation skills.

> *'We don't stop playing because we grow old, we grow old because we stop playing!.'*
> – GEORGE BERNARD SHAW, IRISH PLAYWRIGHT AND POLITICAL ACTIVIST

Emotional Domain

PART 3: RELEASE THE HANDBRAKE AND LET IT GO!

I was on a surfing holiday in Bali with friends in 2018. On the way back, I decided to take an alternative flight path, with a long stopover in Dubai airport, partially due to money and a desire for some alone time after a debaucherous adventure.

Whilst I hung around a slick, shiny-surfaced Dubai airport, I wandered into a shop to buy a Moleskine notebook. I bunkered up in Starbucks with a coffee and started journaling. I decided to let the handbrake off, with an incessant speed that was entirely unexpected. I began by breaking down my earliest childhood memories, working up to the present day. I could not honestly recall what prompted this, but I simply wrote and wrote. Eventually I was half a notepad down, recounting some emotional parts of my past: being bullied in school, my dad's struggles with alcohol, his eventual death, my mum's inability to express how she was feeling, failed relationships and my own relationship with alcohol, drugs and intimacy with women.

The floodgates opened. The tears started to stream down my face as I contemplated my own existence.

Self-consciousness overcame me for a period but dissipated as quickly as it had arrived. I didn't care; I was sobbing like a baby in Starbucks with just a cappuccino to soothe me. Instead of holding back, I continued the deep dive into my soul. I probed for patterns of past failed relationships, my own faults and regrets of my shortcomings. The common denominator in every relationship was me!

I broke down the memories that stood out from my childhood, recounting conversations with friends, family bereavements and significant life events all came sprawling out onto the page – uncensored and raw. At that moment, I decided to seek support: making an appointment with a counsellor to process my past, to confront these emotions and to let go.

If we avoid the difficult conversations today, the shackles of yesterday will bear down on us and hinder our progress moving forward.

APPLICATION TO CLINICAL PRACTICE

It is our role as healthcare professionals to guide patients through times of adversity, pain or injury when emotional regulation is tested (Petrini & Arendt-Nielsen, 2020).

Affective reassurance is a tool to help this process. Affective reassurance is used to connect with a person on an emotional level, through active listening, reflection, validation of their experiences and summarisation of the person's story.

This technique helps a person feel listened to in order to increase self-esteem, self-acceptance and the ability to deal with strong emotions. To effectively connect with a person as therapists, we need to understand the relationship with our own emotions (Fig. 10.2). Reflection on your past or present experiences with these emotions provides a stable platform to offer support for the people you work with.

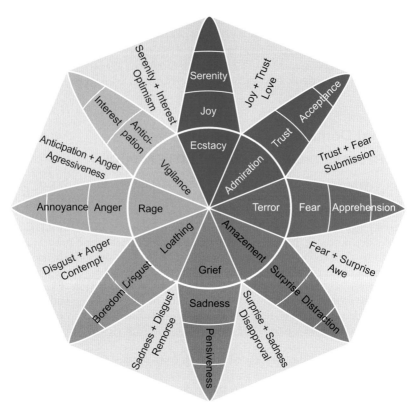

Fig. 10.2 Emotional wheel. (Adapted from Robert Plutchik's Wheel of Emotions. Available at https://commons.wikimedia.org/wiki/File:Plutchik-wheel.svg. Accessed 20 February 2024.)

Mental Domain

PART 4: ACCEPTING THE RAT RACE IN YOUR MIND

'Resilience is strategically managed suffering.'
– ROSS EDGLEY, ATHLETE, ADVENTURER AND AUTHOR, 2020

Every 5 years, in honour of my late dad, I take on a physical or mental challenge that scares the hell out of me. In 2021, a friend and I signed up for the Rat Race Coast to Coast Challenge – a monstrous 105-mile adventure race across the unforgiving Scottish mountains. The race consisted of a 7-mile technical trail run, road cycling, off-road cycling, kayaking and a 14-mile trail run with a 2,500-ft climb at the foot of Ben Nevis, Scotland.

The training preparation was meticulous with periodisation, mindset and nutritional strategies. We felt prepared as we drove up to Scotland with my thoughtful girlfriend as road support. As we arrived at the start point in Nairn, we started to prepare our gear and bikes for the transition point. I was suddenly confronted with a disaster.

I had a broken spoke and my wheel had buckled in the last training ride 1 week previously. I hadn't noticed it as I had been tapering from all forms of training. Panic set in!

We had raised over £3,000 for charity. I was doing it in honour of my dad. My training partner and I had sacrificed countless hours training. The emotion, erratic thoughts and tremors started to run rife throughout my whole body. I couldn't see a solution!

Luckily, my quick-witted girlfriend whom we often joke is led by logic (rather than emotion) quickly and resourcefully switched into action mode as she called our Airbnb host to see if she knew of anyone/anywhere local that might be able to sell me a spare wheel. In a fortuitous twist of fate, our host's son was a semi-professional cyclist and happened to have several bikes lying idle in their garage. The luck of the Irish had struck once again. Our saviour host agreed to provide a wheel for the event bike mechanic to fit and alter as needed.

And so, at 6:00 the following morning, we set off into the coastal Scottish darkness spurred on by our ability to turn around what had initially seemed like a catastrophic situation. My training partner and I had breezed by the 7-mile technical trail run with ease, as we jumped on the bikes, ready to take on the 48-mile road cycle.

Cycling would usually be my strongest discipline. However, at 25 miles, I started to notice an uncharacteristic cramp setting in my thighs. The cramp intensified and it became unbearable as I struggled up the majestic hills of Scotland. Eventually, I was crippled, climbing to the top desperately looking for a suitable hedge to collapse. I was unable to get out of the saddle or even fully extend my leg. The mental chatter became overwhelming!

I repeated the process of climbing a small gradient, gritting my teeth, and painfully searching for somewhere to collapse. After the sixth time sprawling into the ditch, broken, I had started to accept that I may need to withdraw from the race. The same shame and guilt I had experienced in Carlow during my rainy run years earlier began to resurface like an overflowing bath of suppressed emotion.

We moved onto a steep offroad climb with the mind-numbing, excruciating pain in both quadriceps now. We were only around 30 miles into a 105-mile race.

This was suffering and a test of how long I could endure.

I could feel my jaw muscles fatiguing whilst grinding my teeth, refusing to stop.

The pain intensity had ramped up another level. Then an intriguing voice started to repeat in my mind.

'You haven't dealt with Dad passing away! After this race, get some counselling and let it go', the soft alluring voice repeated.

The cramps started to dissipate for a minute as I wrestled with the internal voice. My body was telling me to stop and surrender. My mind was encouraging me to accept and move forward. My heart was compassionately whispering to feel and embrace the sensations rifling through my core.

I had been using mantras during endurance races for several years.

'I am not my body; I am not my mind. I am aware of my body. I am aware of my mind', aggressively repeating this mantra as I come to another steep ascent. The internal screams to seek support and counselling grew louder and more forceful.

Halfway up the hill, I begrudgingly accepted the voice and surrendered. My mind buckled for a minute as I embraced the notion of getting counselling again. I welcomed the feelings of sadness, grief and shame. The cramp gradually subsided in my legs as I learned to nurture the sensations I was experiencing. A lightness consumed my body, as I grew physically stronger.

My mental challenge was manifesting in my body as a physical cramp. I was 34 miles into a 105-mile race after being subjected to one of the most difficult internal battles of my life, in my mind.

After I accepted this, I grew happier, stronger and faster. With each mile, the sensations were embraced with a childlike curiosity, freedom and sense of play. I did not experience any further cramp for the remaining 71 miles.

Rat Race Coast to Coast was completed. I took myself away to a quiet corner after the race following a celebratory drink with my thoughtful girlfriend, training partner and family. I welcomed the emotions as tears of joy began flowing down my cheeks. The tears were different to that autumn evening in Carlow. They had an indescribable warmth and a sweet addictive taste.

I had wrestled with these emotions for years, despite helping others on a weekly basis explore their own pain experiences. I was deflecting my own issues and focusing on others.

The physical challenge of Rat Race was a transformative experience. I had to endure and suffer to fully accept, investigate and nurture the same sensations that crippled me. I had spent years running away from the grief. The rat race was over in my mind – the same race I had been running for over 17 years since Dad passed away.

APPLICATION TO CLINICAL PRACTICE

Mental fitness encapsulates many traits, most of which are exemplified in this story. The ability to think creatively from various perspectives is oftentimes known as mental agility. Within a clinical context, therapists can help a person see their blind spots, reframing the opportunity an injury presents.

Grit is defined, by Angela Duckworth (2017), as the passion and perseverance for long-term goals. The dark side of grit is knowing if persistence with a goal is detrimental or constructive. Endurance athletes provide a great example of a cohort who may be avoiding difficult conversations with themselves yet mastering the physical domain of mental fitness. We are either running away from or towards something more meaningful.

Mental toughness is a broad term, born from the sports performance literature (Jones *et al.*, 2002), comprising hardiness, coping skills, resiliency and optimism (Liew *et al.*, 2019, p. 11). Seligman defines optimism as 'the ability to notice the positive in any situation, refocusing on what they can control and supporting them to take purposeful action'. Optimism serves as a superpower once applied correctly. Setbacks are temporary, local or changeable.

Mental toughness aims to help an individual excel through adversity, whereas resiliency strives to return someone to baseline function despite challenging circumstances.

Mental fitness is a complex interplay of these characteristics. They all have their own distinct sounds, like instruments in a symphony, yet when applied together, they create a beautiful melody to bounce back from the brink. The duty of the therapist is to know the names of these instruments before we decipher how to coach our patients to play them.

Spiritual Domain

PART 5: PIVOT FROM A STABLE BASE

'Easy choice, hard life. Hard choice, easy life.'
– JERZY GREGOREK, WORLD CHAMPION WEIGHTLIFTER, POETRY WRITER AND
THE CO-AUTHOR OF *THE HAPPY BODY*

As a kid, we did not go on family holidays as we had a business to run. In my adulthood, travel and adventure have always been important to me as a result. This meant when I heard other kids talk about family holidays, I was overcome with envy. In 2018, my mum, sisters and their families all agreed we would go on our first family holiday to Lanzarote. I was stoked with excitement!

For many moons, I dreamed of working in pro sport.

I had the opportunity to work with the Great Britain Basketball Under 20 squad between 2013 and 2019, travelling to European championships, working with incredible coaches, diligent therapists and inspiring athletes. I had been building relationships with the Great Britain coaching staff, hoping to be promoted to the senior Great Britain team.

The stable family base was about to be stress tested though.

In January 2018, the Head of Sports Medicine for Great Britain Basketball, Paul Fisher, called. He asked if I was available to come away with the senior Great Britain squad for a training camp in Portugal in February. He gleefully exclaimed that the head coach, Jose 'Chema'

Buceta, had asked specifically for me. I admired 'Chema', who is a psychology professor in Madrid as well as a phenomenal person, coach and mentor. Paul implied that it would likely result in going to the Gold Coast, Australia, for the Commonwealth Games 2018 in March of that year.

I had waited for this opportunity for 5 years and had finally made the grade. I paused with anticipation to find out the details. My heart started to sink as I remembered the upcoming holiday. The Head of Sports Medicine continued with the respective dates of the training camp and the Commonwealth Games.

My fears had been realised. The dates clashed with a skiing trip I had planned with friends to Meribel, France, and to make matters worse, the family holiday clashed with the Commonwealth Games in the Gold Coast, Australia. My heart sank!

The decision was now whether to follow a career path or stick with my values. Earlier that year, I had done some self-development work, reflecting on what is important to me, and defined my personal values – family, adaptable, adventure, growth and curiosity.

The ability to pivot, change direction and be adaptable has served me well in my career. Adaptability is a strong skill to possess as you can flex to the demands of any situation. However, having a strong footing of where you came from and what is most important to you is a life lesson that cannot be overemphasised.

The best stories are the ones which do not have a definitive ending …

What decision would you have made?

APPLICATION TO CLINICAL PRACTICE

Values-based goal setting refers to the will to match our behaviour to our values. We need to understand that the best indicator of future behaviour is our past behaviour. As therapists, we can use our humble enquiry skills to explore a patient's past behaviour when injured and gauge their values from this (Mold, 2017).

Strength of character is one of the most important competencies of resilience. In the above story, the predefined values help steer the decision towards what matters. If you compromise your values once, they are put into question for every decision thereafter (Pincus et al., 2013).

How will you measure your life?

Core values and purpose provide a northern star to orientate yourself towards when difficult decisions arise. This uncertainty may manifest as tension you hold within your body, unsettled mind or a 'gut feeling' something is off. 'Gut feeling' or embodied cognition has been explored in relation to the uncertainty in clinical decision-making (Langridge et al., 2016). This uncertainty will be experienced on a daily basis in clinical practice.

As you advance your career, moving into senior roles, advanced clinical practice or managerial positions, stepping outside of your comfort zone is inevitable. Uncertainty can be managed with a suitable framework (Helou et al., 2020) and a deep understanding of what defines you, your personal values.

'Medicine's ground state is uncertainty; and wisdom – for the patients, therapists, doctors – is defined by how one copes with it.'

ATUL GAWANDE

Healthcare is changing for the better, moving away from the assumption that health is the absence of problems (Mold, 2017).

We will need to reconceptualise mental health into a positive construct, utilising mental fitness, thus preparing the next generation with tools to cope with the future. The PRP helps us understand the application of mental fitness, moving away from the stigmatised mental health terminology of the past. Mental fitness is a potential term to reframe how society views mental health, using resilience as a cornerstone to its implementation.

Resilience is defined as 'the psychological capacity to adapt to stressful situations and bounce back from adverse conditions' (Luthar *et al.*, 2000). It is commonly seen as a positive trait, which it is without doubt. However, there is a negative side to resilience when it is fuelled by denial, avoidance or self-enhancement. This can breed destructive outcomes in sport, at work or at home. The aspirational side of resiliency should be focused on building mental toughness, strong relationships and signature strengths (Seligman *et al.*, 2018).

The stories detailed in this chapter portray the positive and negative aspects of a resilient mind, adapting through the physical, emotional and psychological challenges. Exercise is a magic pill that should be promoted, until it does not serve a healthy cause. Emotional intelligence is clever until we are so smart; we avoid seeking psychological support. Mental toughness is advantageous until it becomes an armour against emotional vulnerability.

If every decision is easy, you are not asking yourself the difficult questions.

The complex interplay of the mind, the body and our emotions dictate how this shift in mental health will be navigated. To effectively guide our patients, we need to understand our own relationship as therapists with change, challenges, strong emotional states and adversity. Turning the lens inwards to focus on our own views of the physical, emotional, mental and spiritual domains will provide the groundwork to guide our patients back to what matters most to them.

Positive psychology and mental fitness have been adopted within schools, computing, corporate business and the military. Yet its application has not been considered within healthcare. Further research into the PERMA Model of Well-Being may offer an answer to shift healthcare towards optimising mental health and fitness.

The PERMA Model focuses on positive emotions, engagement, relationships, meaning and accomplishments (Seligman, 2011). The human condition is complex beyond measure and positive psychology is not a panacea to all health-related issues. Despite this, it may prove to be the psychological first aid that therapists of the future need.

Reflection – Chrystal Lynch

Chrystal Lynch, a physiotherapist from Barbados, shares her personal insights from studying physiotherapy, her own relationship with mental health and advice for aspiring therapists.

When I started my university journey, I was very naïve in my understanding of mental health, mental fitness, resilience and how to effectively face challenges. Whenever mental health was mentioned, terms such as depression, suicide, anxiety and eating disorders, just to name a few, would pop into my mind. I thought these terms didn't apply to me. This is how the society I grew up in presented mental health. When I reached university, I learnt that those were just the tip of the iceberg.

Mental health has to do with every human being, as no one is excluded. It includes our emotional, psychological and social wellbeing. How we act, think and feel throughout every stage of our life. As you can see, these three things, namely emotional (feeling), psychological (thinking) and social (acting), are major aspects that make us human. Just because someone is not showing signs of depression, anxiety or eating disorders does not mean they have good mental fitness.

To be quite honest, I would say those labelled with mental health problems are better at handling the stress and their mental fitness utilising daily coping strategies.

So, how mentally fit are we? Do we have the skills? Am I performing at my best?

I failed my first year of physiotherapy school. To be honest, I was shocked something like that could happen to me. I did try to improve myself during my repeat year after doing some deep reflective work. Being a student, local or overseas, is an incredibly challenging experience. It is even more difficult when you don't have the skills and practices to maintain your state of wellbeing.

Before leaving home to study, many people told me:

'The gap between home and university is huge.'

'You gotta put in more work.'

'You'll be fine once you study.'

So, I just thought, 'I'll be fine once I study hard enough, put in the work and time'. How wrong I was! I am not saying this is the same for everyone. We are all different. I needed the mental practices to work smarter and balance the other components of my wellbeing.

Through a mental health campaign in my second year of university, I was able to build up my mental skill toolbox. It was not easy. I had to find what worked best for me, but it was worth it. It does take discipline to practise daily habits and try others. The results are worth it in the end.

Honestly, leaving university and getting started in the working life is no less stress, just a different arena. I still use these tools to help me navigate my day-to-day routine. I have still not perfected mental fitness and my days can be a rollercoaster blur at times. However, I have got better at handling and manoeuvring through situations that could potentially unsettle my mind.

You're not alone; we are all here fighting along with you, so don't give up!

Five Key Takeaways

1. Mental fitness provides a positive reframing to help us move forwards and past the stigma around mental health.
2. Challenge, control and commitment underpin the concept of mental fitness.
3. Positive psychology and the PERMA Model can help us flourish as clinicians, leading to better outcomes and relationships with our patients.
4. As healthcare professionals, we need to consider our own relationships within certain health domains – physical, mental, emotional, spiritual and social.
5. Optimism, resilience and emotional regulation (notably, self-efficacy and self-compassion) are superpowers to be leveraged to enhance your career. More research is required in these areas.

Five Self-Directed Reflections

1. What inspired you to become a therapist?
2. How will you measure your career?
3. What are you running away from or towards?
4. What challenges have you overcome recently?
5. What domain do you spend the most time working on?

References

De Hert, S. (2020). Burnout in healthcare workers: Prevalence, impact and preventative strategies. *Local and Regional Anaesthesia, 13*, 171–183. https://doi.org/10.2147/LRA.S240564.

Duckworth, A. (2017). *Grit: The power of passion and perseverance* (1st ed.). Vermilion.

Edgley, R. (2020). *The art of resilience: Strategies for an unbreakable mind and body* (1st ed., p. 223). HarperCollins Publishers.

Helou, M., DiazGranados, D., Ryan, S., & Cyrus, J. (2020). Uncertainty in decision making in medicine: A scoping review and thematic analysis of conceptual models. *Academic Medicine, 95*(1), 157–165. https://doi.org/10.1097/ACM.0000000000002902.

Henderson, M., Madan, I., & Hotopf, M. (2014). Work and mental health in the UK. *British Medical Journal, 348*, g2256. https://doi.org/10.1136/bmj.g2256.

Jones, G., Hanton, S., & Connaughton, D. (2002). What is this thing called mental toughness? An investigation of elite sport performers. *Journal of Applied Sport Psychology, 14*(3), 205–218. https://doi.org/10.1080/10413200290103509.

Kandola, A. (2020). Individual and combined associations between cardiorespiratory fitness and grip strength with common mental disorders: A prospective cohort study in the UK Biobank. *BMC Medicine, 18*, 303. https://doi.org/10.1186/s12916-020-01782-9.

Langridge, N., Roberts, L., & Pope, C. (2016). The role of clinician emotion in clinical reasoning: Balancing the analytical process. *Manual Therapy, 21*, 277–281. https://doi.org/10.1016/j.math.2015.06.007.

Liew, G., Kuan, G., Chin, N., & Hashim, H. A. (2019). Mental toughness in sport: Systematic review and future directions. *German Journal of Exercise and Sport Research, 49*(4), 11.

Luthar, S., Cicchetti, D., & Becker, B. (2000). The construct of resilience: A critical evaluation and guidelines for future work. *Child Development, 71*(3), 543–562. https://doi.org/10.1111/1467-8624.00164.

Mold, J. (2017). Goal-directed health care: Redefining health and health care in the era of value-based care. *Cureus, 9*(2), e1043. https://doi.org/10.7759/cureus.1043.

Pelletier, L., Shamila, S., Scott, B., & Demers, A. (2017). Self-management of mood and/or anxiety disorders through physical activity/exercise. *Health Promotion and Chronic Disease Prevention in Canada: Research, Policy, and Practice, 37*(5), 27–32.

Petrini, L., & Arendt-Nielsen, L. (2020). Understanding pain catastrophising: Putting the pieces together. *Frontiers in Psychology, 11*, 603420. https://doi.org/10.3389/fpsyg.2020.603420.

Pincus, T., Holt, N., Vogel, S., Underwood, M., Savage, R., Walsh, D., & Taylor, S. (2013). Cognitive and affective reassurance and patient outcomes in primary care: A systematic review. *Pain, 154*(11), 2407–2416. https://doi.org/10.1016/j.pain.2013.07.019.

Seligman, M. (2011). *Flourish: A new understanding of happiness and well-being – how to achieve them* (pp. 152–177). London: Nicholas Brealey Publishing.

Seligman, M., Schwartz, T., Bennis, W., & Thomas, R. (2018). *On mental toughness*. London: Harvard Business Review.

Whitebread, A., Coltman, P., Jameson, H., & Lander, R. (2009). Play, cognition, and self-regulation: What exactly are children learning when they learn through play? *Educational and Child Psychology, 26*(2), 40–52.

Further Reading

de Bot, C., Boemaars, C., & Dierx, J. (2019). Positive health as a new concept for physiotherapy in the Netherlands? *European Public Health Conference, 29*(4). https://doi.org/10.1093/eurpub/ckz186.200.

Elphinston, R. A., Sterling, M., Kenardy, J., Smeets, R., & Armfield, N. R. (2020). The mechanisms of effect of a physiotherapist-delivered integrated psychological and exercise intervention for acute whiplash-associated disorders: Secondary mediation analysis of a randomized control trial. *Pain Reports, 5*(5), e835. https://doi.org/10.1097/PR9.0000000000000835.

Karel, Y., Van Vliet, M., Lugtigheid, C., De Bot, C., & Dierx, J. (2019). The concept of positive health for students/lecturers in the Netherlands. *International Journal of Health Promotion and Education, 57*(5), 286–296. https://doi.org/10.1080/14635240.2019.1623707.

Karimova, H. (2022). *The emotion wheel: What is it and how to use it.* Available at https://positivepsychology.com/emotion-wheel/. Accessed 17 October 2022.

Linn, M. (2017). A study on the relationship of hardiness and psychological stress responses. *Yadanabon University Research Journal, 8*(1), 2.

Mohatashami, A., Tajari, F., & Rad, M. (2015). Studying the relationship between hardiness and resilience personality traits and academic achievement among students of Kashan University in 2014. *Cumhuriyet Science Journal, 36*, 3294–3301.

Norris, M., & Wainwright, E. (2022). Learning professional touch: An exploration of pre-registration physiotherapy students' experiences. *Physiotherapy Theory and Practice, 38*(1), 90–100. https://doi.org/10.1080/09593985.2020.1725944.

Penn Positive Psychology Centre. (2022). *Resilience – skill-set.* The Trustees of the University of Pennsylvania. Available at https://ppc.sas.upenn.edu/resilience-programs/resilience-skill-set. Accessed 17 October 2022.

Willink, J., & Babin, L. (2015). *Extreme ownership: How US Navy seals lead and win.* New York: St. Martin's Press.

CHAPTER 11

High Performance – Leading Yourself and Others With Purpose

David Cosgrave ■ Federico Picchetti

> 'High performance means true confidence, understanding what happens around me. If the environment changes, I will figure it out.'
> – Rich Diviney, retired Navy SEAL and founder of the Attributes,
> as quoted on *Sleep Eat Perform Repeat* podcast, 2021

CHAPTER OUTLINE

Introduction
Federico's Story
High Performance
Meaningfulness
Need Fulfilment
Belongingness
Purpose

What Could Federico's Elevator Pitch Sound Like?
Try It for Yourself
Leading Yourself With Purpose
Five Key Takeaways
Five Self-Directed Reflections

Introduction

What does the term high performance mean to you?

I challenge you to come up with a catchy answer.

It could be the easiest interview, the ultimate door opener or the one-in-a-million opportunity that all young practitioners strive for. I call this 'the elevator pitch'. You will be surprised how hard it is to define the concept of high performance with clarity. It encompasses so much, has so many tangents and is obtuse but needs to be sharp.

It is something that is easier to describe when it is absent, a concept that makes it peculiarly like culture.

I like to describe it as all the things we do in our environment that give us a chance to be a little bit better, or luckier, than the other guys.

Now that we have a description of high performance, let's investigate how we might lead ourselves and other high-performers with purpose. In this chapter I am going to walk you through some concepts that are hard to describe but will seem quite common. You will be surprised how hard it is to explain the 'Who am I?' and 'Why am I here?' questions about life. It will be demanding to zone in on the levers that motivate you and the deep, formative needs that should be achieved for you to feel fulfilled. Finally, I must remind you that we are social creatures, and the perception of finding your community is so galvanising that everyone strives to belong to something a bit bigger than themselves.

Federico's Story

FEDERICO IS AN ITALIAN PHYSIOTHERAPIST WHO KNOWS ABOUT HIGH PERFORMANCE; HERE IS HIS JOURNEY

I was a young footballer playing in a professional youth academy. I had two bad knee injuries when I was 16 years old that kept me out of football for 8 months. Then unfortunately I had another surgery 3 years later. This experience helped me understand the rehab process and how athletes and clients can feel. It also opened Pandora's box of worries, anxiety and pain.

FEDERICO EXPERIENCED A HIGH PERFORMANCE ENVIRONMENT AS A PLAYER AND AS A PRACTITIONER

Now that I am a physiotherapist, I know it is essential that I help my athletes set their goals, listen to them on bad days, motivate them, include them in the programming and facilitate a successful return to play or return to normal life for them.

THERE IS NOW A DEEPER MEANINGFULNESS TO FEDERICO'S PROFESSIONAL IDENTITY

When I started as a physiotherapist my goals were simple: study books, train what I learn and emulate senior practitioners I looked up to. The more I learned, the more I felt empowered, and then, in turn, I grew. At first, the process was gradual, and in an unconscious manner I became more confident. Then more consciously I became aware of what I believed in. I had found meaningfulness in my work and understood who I was.

WHEN WORK DOESN'T FEEL LIKE A CHORE

I tend to absorb so much knowledge that my peers jokingly say to me, 'You are a sponge, my friend'. When work and learning seem like joy, I do not struggle to find motivation. Every day I gain energy and motivation watching my athletes get stronger as I lead them through the rehabilitation process, knowing that I played a big role.

BEING THERE FOR THE ATHLETE FULFILS AN IMPORTANT NEED FOR FEDERICO

I like challenges, and I like the feeling of victory. When you work with an athlete in a team, you can have the emotions that they have during the game. Their victory is your victory. If they feel it, you can make a big change in their career. You gain trust – they start to follow you, to be more motivated, reaching their goals and fulfilling their potential.

WORKING COLLABORATIVELY WITH OTHER EXPERTS CREATES A SPECIAL BELONGINGNESS

There are so many different people who support the process, for example, doctors, coaches, managers, athletic trainers, chiropractors and general managers. We are all different people, in different departments and with different goals for the club, but we all unite to lead the players as we try to secure a win, a trophy or a championship. If altogether you make the right decision, it will be a win for the player, practitioner, person, team and club.

AND FINALLY, WHY DOES HE DO IT?

I am here to help. I am a servant to those athletes who need me. I believe that you should do what you really love because you put more passion into it and feel more happiness every day. I have found my purpose and it has told me to do what I really love: helping athletes.

Federico's story gives us a great insight into concepts around meaningfulness, motivation, need fulfilment, belonging and the big purposeful question of 'Why am I here?' Using it as a framework, we can try to answer some of these existential questions for ourselves and find a path towards our own individual purpose (see Chapter 2).

High Performance

Our environment demands high standards, personal accountability, shared ownership of a task and a zoomed-out view of the bigger picture that guides us.

This is often called the North Star, a light in the distance. It's never truly within our reach but it is reassuring to know we're moving towards our destination.

You may have heard the African proverb, 'If you want to go fast, go alone. If you want to go far, go together'. This is another essential component of high performance. You can be a high-performer but still need others to release the potential within high performance.

So many medical professionals of physiotherapy, manual therapy and strength coaching work alone as high-performers and strive to find a group or team of athletes that share this passion for high performance. Federico has found this and collaborates with experts to find the gains that may keep them one step ahead of their rivals.

Meaningfulness

'Who am I?' This seems like a simple question, but it is the trickiest of trick questions! The answer, however, becomes clearer the older we get. Over time, our self-identity becomes more secure as we face experiences that test our beliefs and value systems.

Understanding what events in life affect our feelings and drive our behaviours allows us to place energy into activities and individuals that reward the investment. This understanding of oneself creates a self-awareness that promotes motivation to further explore the meaning in life and the quest to find purpose.

As is so common in altruistic professions like physiotherapy, there can be a feeling that the meaningful work being done is a calling and the self-identity of the person and practitioner can become one. In Federico's story it is clear that he feels a vocational calling to be a physiotherapist and identifies with pride in his professional title.

Need Fulfilment

We have all heard of Maslow's hierarchy of needs. It may not stand up to academic scrutiny, but it is a useful model when trying to understand motivation. Our primitive physiological needs such as hunger, thirst and safety are easily met without the complications of famine, drought and wild animals in the modern era.

More personal and complex needs like love, belonging and esteem-boosting work motivate us to behave in certain ways to fulfil and meet these intrinsic needs. Understanding the environment and landscape we find ourselves in presents us with many motivational levers to pull. Knowing that we can find food, water and friendship in our environment fulfils us and motivates us with positive intent.

Some of the rewards we seek can also be extrinsically fulfilling, like winning a game or a trophy, as mentioned in Federico's story.

Belongingness

The motivation to belong to something bigger than us is central to our existence. We start in our family unit, move to friendship groups and school teams and soon find our community and social tribe. We all have an inherent need for an affiliation to a social group that helps describe who we are and sometimes who we are not.

While seeming like a physical construct, the perception of belonging is as powerful as being in the presence of others, as unpacked in the wonderful book by Owen Eastwood, *Belonging: The Ancient Code of Togetherness* (2022). Being a member of a group and identifying with other members has associated geographically diverse groups for centuries, but now the availability of online groups is a phenomenal development in belongingness in the modern era.

From Federico's account you can sense the pride he feels in being part of the physiotherapy community, and his perception of belonging to this group motivates him to serve those that need his care.

Purpose

The complex question 'Why am I here?' does not always need to be answered. By simply asking the question you are checking in with yourself to see if what you are doing is right and if the activity is worthwhile and rewarding to your value system. To be purposeful and work with purpose demonstrates that an individual is basing their actions on values that they have predefined as drivers of their behaviour.

A person can find purpose in their life, their work or the greater society. When a person finds their purpose, their mission becomes to influence others to find theirs. The athletes Federico works with become motivated to develop their own goals, bypass them and find meaning in their injury or rehabilitation. Federico's personal purpose, informed by his own experience of injury, is to help athletes overcome worry, anxiety and pain.

What Could Federico's Elevator Pitch Sound Like?

I am a proud physiotherapist who has experienced career-ending injuries during my football career. Instead of letting these injuries define my self-identity, I have used them to give meaning to my life as a physiotherapist and fulfil my need to serve and help athletes purposefully on their own journeys.

Try It for Yourself

I am a (*belonging*) that has experienced (*meaning*) during my life. Instead of letting this (*life-defining event*) define my self-identity (*who I am*), I have used it to (*why am I here*) and fulfil my need to (*need fulfilment*) and (*personal purpose*).

Leading Yourself With Purpose

Having reviewed Federico's story we can see that he was very clear about how he led himself with purpose. But what about leading others?

Before you can lead others, you must first lead yourself. Know thyself, know thy team and grow thy team is a go-to when discussing the importance of self-awareness with leaders. Leading with purpose involves setting common value-based goals, staying focused in the choppy seas of collaboration and motivating yourself and your team to achieve those common goals in a harmonious and safe environment.

To lead yourself with purpose, you must first define your own personal mission, vision and values. These are the guiding principles that will help you make decisions and take actions aligned with your purpose. You must also set clear goals for yourself and develop a plan to achieve them. This requires discipline, focus and persistence. I recommend doing this as an exercise.

As with anything in high performance, you need to find what works for you. There is some depth to these takeaways, so take your time and make sense of them for yourself.

Five Key Takeaways

1. Key principles for leading yourself

   Self-awareness: Understand your strengths and weaknesses. Document your core values, beliefs and motivations to ensure effective self-leadership before concentrating on others.

   Clarity of purpose: Define your personal mission, vision and values, and set clear goals for yourself that align with them.

   Focus and discipline: Stay focused on your goals and maintain discipline to take consistent action towards achieving them.

   Continuous learning and improvement: Develop a growth mindset and invest in your own learning and development. Seek out feedback and actively seek to improve your skills and knowledge.

   Resilience: Develop the resilience to overcome setbacks and failures and stay focused on your goals in the face of challenges.

   Self-care: Take care of your physical, emotional and mental wellbeing, and maintain a healthy work-life balance.

   Accountability: Take responsibility for your actions and decisions and hold yourself accountable for achieving your goals.

   By following these principles, you can effectively lead yourself towards personal and professional success.

2. Tools to develop self-awareness

   Understanding your strengths and weaknesses on the journey of discovery is a crucial aspect of effective leadership. Before you can lead others, you must first lead yourself. To do that it is essential for you to do the work and develop your self-awareness.

   Using these tools, you can fast-track your self-awareness:

   Online personality assessments: While often lacking scientific reliability, these easy-to-use tools can give you insights that allow dialogue with others about how you see yourself and how they see you.

   360-Degree feedback: This involves pooling feedback from a trusted confidante about your behaviour and characteristics. While uncomfortable, this exercise can give valuable insights into your blind spots as perceived by others.

   Journaling: Writing down events and your feelings is a powerful tool when reflecting. Dissecting these experiences can shine a light on your thinking and the narrative you tell yourself.

   Mindfulness: Trying to be present in your body through intentional presence, meditation and breathing exercises allows you to control your environment and regulate your emotions.

Executive coaching: Engaging the service of an expert coach creates accountability and support during lonely phases of leadership.

3. How to find your core values (see Chapter 2)

Core values change over time. It's tricky to know if they've changed, so learning how to document your core values is a fantastic skill. Discovering your core values can help you clarify what drives you and support your decision-making in all areas of your life.

Use these simple steps to identify your core values:

Reflect on your life experiences so far: When were you at your happiest? Think about the times when you felt most fulfilled. What values were present in those experiences? Document the big events and how you got there.

Identify your role models: Who are the people you respect? What are the values you admire in them? How do you embody the values of your role model in your own behaviour?

What gets you out of bed in the morning? List the daily tasks that energise you. What experiences have made you feel alive? What values are present and who are the people you are sharing the experiences with?

Sacred values: What values do you believe to be unbreakable? Rank the importance of the core values and clarify values that have not changed as your identity has grown.

Back-test your beliefs: Are your core values congruent with how you see the world? Test them by applying them to different areas of your life and the story you tell yourself.

By reflecting on your values, you ensure you are making decisions that align with your internal compass.

4. Leading others with purpose

To lead others with purpose, they must see the good in your actions and have faith in your value system. The followers will feel part of your tribe and their perception of belonging will fulfil their inherent desire to belong. Therefore, as a leader you must create a shared vision and mission that inspires your team to work towards a common goal. You must communicate this vision clearly and motivate your team to act towards achieving it. This involves creating a culture of high performance where everyone is focused on delivering exceptional results and constantly improving.

Here are some key principles for leading yourself and others with purpose:

Define your purpose: Clarify your personal mission, vision and values, and set clear goals for yourself.

Focus on your strengths: Identify your strengths and focus on developing them further. Build a team around you that complements your strengths and compensates for your weaknesses.

Act: Turn your goals into action by developing a plan, staying focused and taking consistent action towards achieving them.

Be resilient: High performance requires resilience. Stay focused on your goals and don't let setbacks or failures derail you. Use failures as learning opportunities and keep pushing forward.

Inspire others: Create a shared vision and mission that inspires your team to work towards a common goal. Communicate this vision clearly and motivate your team to act towards achieving it.

Develop others: Invest in the development of your team members and create opportunities for them to grow and succeed. Build a culture of continuous learning and improvement.

Lead by example: As a leader, you must lead by example. Model the behaviours and values that you want your team to exhibit and hold yourself and others accountable for delivering exceptional results.

5. High performance is a never-ending quest. Enjoy the ride!

I hope you have enjoyed reading this chapter and have taken plenty of notes. Please try the takeaway sections to help you identify the motivational drivers that support your behaviour, mould your identity and secure your place in the tribe you feel safe in – as you go about your purposeful work.

Five Self-Directed Reflections

1. Which principles for leading yourself stand out for you?
2. How can you improve your self-awareness starting today?
3. Can you now clearly articulate your values? Would these match up with non-negotiable behaviours?
4. Can you inspire, develop and lead more?
5. What does high performance mean to you, as defined by the podcast *Sleep Eat Perform Repeat*?

References

Diviney, R. (2021). *The attributes: 25 hidden drivers of optimal performance.* Virgin Books, as quoted from the podcast *Sleep Eat Perform Repeat.*

Eastwood, O. (2022). *Belonging: Unlock your potential with the Ancient Code of Togetherness.* Quercus.

CHAPTER 12

Life/Work Alignment

Mary O'Keefe ■ Barbara Sanders

'Rather than balance, I believe in alignment.'
Dr. Michael Gervais, host of the Finding Mastery podcast, high-performance sports psychologist and co-founder of 'Compete to Create', as quoted on the 'Sleep Eat Perform Repeat' podcast

Introduction

This chapter will explore the concept of life/work alignment for sports physiotherapists, focusing on the specific challenges we face and potential methods we can employ to achieve balance and wellbeing. As two physiotherapists who have experience working in highly demanding sports settings – spending more time imbalanced than balanced and misaligned than the 'ideal' and elusive 'aligned' – we aim to steer clear of patronising statements and farfetched solutions.

We wish to be upfront from the get-go: Being a sports physiotherapist is no picnic. It can be incredibly fun and rewarding, and the rushes of the wins and losses are immense, but it is not synonymous with life/work alignment, particularly at elite levels. It involves long hours, emotional labour, intensive communication, high levels of responsibility and quick decisions. It can be difficult too depending on life stage: early career, mid-career and family responsibilities, late career and planning for retirement and adapting to life transitions and events. Life and work are a constant juggling act for the sports physiotherapist.

We hope this chapter has something in it for both the student (or novice) and experienced physiotherapist. We attempt to draw on our own personal experiences, the experiences of other physiotherapists and the literature where relevant. Overall, our chapter can be seen as both a critique and praise of the goal to achieve life/work alignment.

What Is Life/Work Alignment?

Life/work alignment has been defined as the process of harmoniously integrating and balancing the various aspects of one's personal and work life in a way that facilitates overall wellbeing, satisfaction and success. It is different to the work-life balance, which refers to an equal distribution of time and commitment between work and personal life. Life/work alignment strives towards the integration and synergy between work and personal life. Achieving such alignment means your work and personal life complement and support each other, rather than causing unnecessary stress or conflict. I think this would be a physiotherapist's version of nirvana! Key ingredients include the following:

- *Boundary setting:* This includes designated work hours, avoiding work-related activities during personal time and not letting personal issues interfere with work. As a sports physiotherapist, even with the hardest of efforts, is this realistic for most of us? Our work hours are long, often unpredictable. We are constantly connected to the team and athletes. We are human – what is going on in our personal life has large potential to influence how we perform in our work life.

- *Priority setting:* Establishing clear priorities and determining what is truly important in both your personal and professional life. As a physiotherapist, I find this to be quite vague and prescriptive. We all have personal and professional priorities, but setting them doesn't always equal alignment.

- *Time management:* Effectively managing your time to ensure that you can focus on the most important tasks and activities in both your work and personal life. Again, this would be wonderful. But what advice do we give a physiotherapist who is on duty 7 days a week and is the first to arrive and last to leave work?

- *Flexibility:* Being open to adjusting your work and personal routines as needed, to maintain balance and accommodate changes in your life. Sports physiotherapists are experts in flexibility as they constantly must work around team and athlete schedules.

- *Self-awareness:* Understanding your own needs, values, and goals and taking steps to ensure that your work and personal life are aligned with these. When I (Mary) was working in highly stressful environments, I was fully aware that I was stressed and not having the time for my personal life that I should have been having. But acting on that awareness is a different concept. Also, passionate sports physiotherapists – loving thy sport so to speak – need to make sacrifices to improve their knowledge – and so work takes precedence at certain times.

- *Self-care:* Prioritising your physical, mental and emotional wellbeing and taking the necessary steps to maintain your health and reduce stress. Sports physiotherapists are all aware of the importance of self-care – be it exercise, sleep, diet, stress management and so forth. We strive for self-care in all our athletes. For physiotherapists who do not at least attempt to make time for these, it is a good place to start. But, as we can say from experience, self-care is not a magic button you can press. Exercise, sleep, diet and so on can take major hits during times of intense travel with teams and rising injury lists with strong potential to influence the team's success. No one lives in a vacuum. Sports physiotherapists are part of a team.

- *Communication:* Effectively communicating with your employer, co-workers, friends and family about your needs, expectations, and boundaries, to foster understanding and support. Sports physiotherapists must be masters of effective communication – with coaches, other medical staff and of course the athletes. Effectively communicating our expectations and boundaries is reasonable and would be fantastic where relevant, but in many cases, this is not possible.

As you can see, many of the tenets of life/work alignment create issues for sports physiotherapists because of the nature of our work. This means providing generic advice around self-care and resilience in this chapter would be fruitless.

Why Is Life/Work Alignment an Important Skill for Sports Physiotherapists?

While we have been sceptical so far about how realistic it is for sports physiotherapists to achieve life/work alignment, this does not mean that it is not worth striving for. Honing this skill is particularly important given the literature that highlights the levels of burnout that can be experienced by sports physiotherapists. Feeling burned out can lead to poor mental health (e.g., feelings of depression, anxiety and emotional exhaustion); reduced work productivity (feeling burned out can impair physiotherapists' ability to provide effective care to athletes and communicate across the team, which could result in suboptimal treatment outcomes); and lower life and work satisfaction, which can lead to increased turnover and a higher likelihood of leaving the profession altogether. A worrying trend is the number of physiotherapists leaving the profession within 5 years of graduating. This is not specific to sports physiotherapists, but it is something we need to monitor and investigate.

Sports physiotherapists face a number of challenges on a regular basis that leave them susceptible to burnout and could benefit from more attention to life/work alignment:

- *High expectations:* Working with athletes, sports physiotherapists can feel pressured to return to competition quickly after an injury. This is particularly apparent in nonprofessional set-ups, where the knowledge of injury and rehabilitation required is limited. This pressure can come from athletes themselves, coaches or other members of the team. Balancing the need to help athletes recover and return to play with the importance of tissue healing times and proper rehabilitation can be challenging. Further, the broad scientific literature demonstrates that the public and patients, including athletes, hold certain beliefs about injury, pain, and the role of physiotherapy. As a physiotherapist leaving university, I felt completely ill-equipped to deal with this. What is the mainstream in physiotherapy courses now – the downsides of manual therapy, the biopsychosocial model – to name two large shifts in teaching – do not always match what is expected by our athletes. We have the team and athlete expectations, but also our internal expectations of what it means to be performing as a good physiotherapist. There is a mismatch here. If we cannot explain with confidence what we do, and why what we do is important, we are in trouble. Personally, I feel this is a crisis happening in identity where physiotherapists question their relevance. This is quite sad to see, when perhaps less competent professionals can fill our space.

- *Unsocial hours and travel:* Long hours and travel are required to maximally support a team. But these facets of our work life also disrupt personal routines (e.g., sleep, exercise, diet) and strain personal relationships.

- *Emotional stress:* Physiotherapists spend long periods of time with athletes, and while we must work within our scope of practice, we sometimes feel we also operate like counsellors and psychologists – providing the support and encouragement through the injury and rehabilitation process. Supporting athletes through the highs and lows of their careers, from overcoming pains and injuries to celebrating victories, can cultivate deep relationships but also expose physiotherapists to emotional stress. Strong social support from physiotherapists has also been found to help athletes adopt a more positive outlook on their way to recovery. A strong athlete–physiotherapist relationship is necessary for effective treatment and shaping of athletes' expectations of injury rehabilitation, but this can be difficult to achieve.

- *High-pressure, uncomfortable environments:* You will need to make quick decisions, you will be challenged, you will disappoint players and teams, you will be wrong, you will be right but told you are wrong. You could lose your job and be blamed for player recovery or lack of recovery. This all goes with the territory of being a physiotherapist and is to some extent nonmodifiable.

- *Keeping up to date with research and social media:* The field of sports physiotherapy is constantly evolving, which means that you will need to stay up to date with the latest research and techniques. This is very beneficial and fundamental to on-going learning and professional development. But there is a dark side: when opinion is communicated as research. Hello Twitter. There is nothing more nauseating than coming home from a day or a week away of working with a team on complex injury or pain presentations requiring careful and timely communication to go online and see the latest post about how sports physiotherapists are behind the times and need to do different treatments, use different assessment tools and so on. These recommendations are often touted in the absence of any new evidence that they are superior to what we currently do. It drives a combined sense of frustration and guilt all in one moment. You never feel like you know enough. Chasing the latest research – while a necessary part of the job, and much of it can be fantastic – can be detrimental to our mental health if it is communicated from an ivory tower and without context.

- *Communicating with different personalities:* Being a good communicator and creating an effective interaction with an athlete and team is probably the most underestimated skill of being a physiotherapist. Again, we leave our university courses bereft of such skills. Being in constant communication with athletes and teams is very demanding, and in the modern era of advancing technology, we are never off. We are on 24/7, ready to take any questions or queries from our team.

- *Lack of control and autonomy:* Depending on the team environment, one can feel little to no control over one's work environment and the decisions to make. Club culture and the beliefs of the wider management team and squad can influence how competent you feel. This can lead to feelings of frustration and helplessness, which can contribute to burnout.

Life/Work Alignment in Sports Physiotherapy – Fact or Myth?

The answer probably lies in between. The notion of life/work balance has been getting increasing traction over the last few decades. Like many things in life, there is a commercial side to this, with simple life alignment hacks marketed as the solution to the stress and anxiety that come with balancing a demanding career and personal life.

The idea of life/work alignment might be seen as an oversimplification of complex, dynamic, individual circumstances. Sports physiotherapists, like all professionals, have different preferences, needs and priorities, and promoting a one-size-fits-all approach to life/work balance can seem dismissive of these differences.

Life/work alignment can be difficult to achieve when sports physiotherapists – particularly early-career physiotherapists – have limited control over their work schedules or demands. Placing the responsibility on the individual physiotherapist to get aligned or show resilience in the face of stress is ignorant to the wider systemic realities: overwork, inflexible schedules or toxic workplace.

For very busy sports physiotherapists, the idea of achieving a perfect balance between life and work can be far-fetched and unrealistic. If life/work alignment is touted for everyone, it may create a sense of guilt or failure for those physiotherapists who struggle to achieve it.

Sports physiotherapists, like many of us in the year 2023, have blurred boundaries. Technological advances have made it increasingly difficult to separate work and life, with sports physiotherapists often feeling constantly connected to their jobs through WhatsApp team groups and similar. Is it a personal failure to struggle with these blurred boundaries?

Some sports physiotherapists may consciously choose to prioritise their career over other aspects of their life at various times for various reasons, such as career progression, love of their career or financial stability. Is this a problem? For these physiotherapists, advocating life/work alignment hacks could be seen as patronising because it disregards the physiotherapist's agency in making these choices.

How to Move Towards Feelings of Life/Work Alignment

As described, the meaning of life/work alignment may vary from physiotherapist to physiotherapist, or indeed may be deemed unrealistic at certain times. However, there is no denying the benefits to be derived from having a good personal and work life – enriched with meaning. This can result in better mental and physical health, improved relationships and increased job satisfaction and productivity. While it may be difficult to achieve a perfect balance, striving for a healthier balance can have significant benefits.

The following strategies reflect common recommendations for achieving alignment, while others are tailored to the reality of being a sports physiotherapist.

- *Be compassionate towards yourself:* Good sports physiotherapists are athlete and team focused. This can come at the expense of their own needs and health. Recognise the complexities of your job and have compassion towards yourself on bad days and losses – the days when you feel like giving up or feel inadequate. It is part of the territory and knowing this can prepare you for these feelings. If we had known this earlier in our career, we would have been less surprised by the lows.

- *Maintain your physical and emotional wellbeing where possible:* Sports physiotherapists do not need to be lectured on the importance of lifestyle and healthful behaviours. Where possible, ensure you are getting enough physical activities, engaging in hobbies you enjoy, getting enough sleep and good nutrition and spending time with loved ones and friends. These activities may be in disarray from time to time, but try to get back to them where possible, and again be compassionate with yourself.

- *Communicate expectations and boundaries where possible:* In certain environments, one may feel more or less comfortable to communicate their needs for certain work hours, what they can and cannot achieve – and in what timeframes – for an athlete. This is best achieved in collaboration with a supportive team who share consistent messages with their athletes about pain and injury.

- *Avoid social media that hampers your thinking or mood:* If each time you log on to Twitter, Facebook and Instagram, you feel frustrated, anxious or annoyed, it would be wise to rethink your use. This can be difficult for physiotherapists as they are often very dedicated to continuous professional development and wish to keep up with the latest research. But maybe ask yourself, is Twitter and other social media the best way to do this? If it makes you feel good, continue. If not, maybe it is time for that 'digital detox'. I have done this at certain periods of high uncertainty, and I've found it helpful.

- *Build a support network:* Having bad days, feeling incompetent and feeling like an imposter are not desirable but are common experiences among sports physiotherapists. This is exacerbated by the criticisms of physiotherapy – and its value – from actual physiotherapists. It can be easy to feel lost. It can be helpful to talk to like-minded people in your profession about cases, struggles and so on. This could be setting up a group of sports physiotherapists with an interest in a certain sport (e.g., rowing, soccer, boxing) and certain pain/injuries (e.g., tendinopathy, back pain) and setting a plan to meet at certain times or having a message board/group. When I was struggling with deep feelings of uncertainty – what's the point of being a physiotherapist, I am useless and so on – discussing this within a supportive network was helpful to my confidence.

- *Expecting – and planning for – periods of higher stress:* Setting yourself up to avoid stress and have the perfect life/work balance will set you up for failure. Once you find yourself in a very busy and stressful situation, you may become overwhelmed. Accepting that there are periods of feeling busy and highly stressful is the first step to putting a plan in place for how you can cope. Communication with people in your personal life about upcoming stresses can also keep everybody in the loop about changing situations.

- *Respect your clinical experience:* Clinical experience is an often forgotten component of delivering evidence-based patient-centred care. It is not all about systematic reviews and what popular physiotherapists recommend on Twitter. We must not forget this. Appraise all new research claims of treatment ineffectiveness and effectiveness critically. Assess the communicator of these claims. How trustworthy are they? Are the research recommendations being applied broadly, without reflecting individual complex patient presentations? Respect the research – some are fantastic, but some are outright awful – so do not be a slave to it.
- *Flexibility and creativity:* Feeling life/work alignment balance may require some creativity and flexibility. For example, some people may be able to negotiate flexible work hours to better align with personal needs and priorities. Others may find ways to incorporate personal interests into their work, such as taking on projects that align with personal passions.

Inspiration From Barbara Sanders – A Book That Changed Her Life

Dr. Stephen Covey wrote the book *The 7 Habits of Highly Effective People* in 1989. Since that time there have been more than 40 million copies sold and it has been published in 40 languages (Covey, 1997). It is the best-selling nonfiction book in history. I became a facilitator for the 20-hour course in 2002 after attending one of the workshops offered at our university. Since that time, Covey's common-sense approach has become routine to me. Dr. Covey takes some basic principles and organises them to help individuals build character, not just to achieve success. After reading, studying, discussing and teaching for decades, he was able to synthesise his thoughts and convey them so that a wide variety of readers could understand. His major approach was to instil discipline through character. It is now 2023 and his words of wisdom endure. In the coming chapter, I will try to highlight each habit and how I have incorporated it into my leadership.

Covey talks about the concepts of personality vs character using the illustration of an iceberg to help us grasp his intent. Personality is what we see above the water; character is that very large chunk of ice that we do not see under the water. Too often personality is what attracts us to others, and we fail to see the underlying character. Character is who we are and communicates far more than anything we say or do. He also describes the concepts of paradigms and how we often need to make a paradigm shift. We can describe paradigms as a map through which we see the territory ahead of us. To get somewhere, we need to best map; without it, even with our best efforts to move we would be lost. Our actions have nothing to do with behaviour or attitude unless we have the right map. Our mental maps are how we see things, our lens, so to speak. If we have the wrong mental map, our actions may lead to the wrong outcomes. Changing our mental map is what Covey describes as a paradigm shift … the 'Aha!' moment. Our character comes through when we can shift our paradigms and thus perhaps our habits. Habits are our consistent and often unconscious behaviour patterns. Covey tells us that habit is the intersection of knowledge, skill and desire. Knowledge is theoretical, knowing what to do and why. Skill is how we do it. And desire is the motivation, the want to do.

The 7 Habits are not a specific guide on how to, but a way to think about how we approach our life – how we think, how we are motivated and what we do. Covey tells us that the 7 Habits are habits of effectiveness – they are based on principles and become the basis of our character.

HABIT 1 – BE PROACTIVE

Habit 1 is the habit of personal vision – the thought that our behaviour is based on our decision, and we have the freedom to make our decisions. For instance, our paradigm may let someone 'push our buttons', but we can change that by thinking about why an action leads to our response. Instead of immediate response, take time, think and decide on the best response. Covey describes this as being proactive and not reactive. Think of the stimulus-response paradigm. If we fail to choose, we are reactive. Another concept in this habit is the use of our efforts and time. They should be directed towards things we can influence and not things we cannot. Covey calls this the circle of influence vs the circle of concern.

The circle of concern includes things that we have no control over or at least little control. The circle of influence includes those things that we have direct or indirect control over. No control problems are those that we should just accept and not focus on or let control us. For instance, the traffic in the city where I lived for years was just horrible; it could take hours to go only a few miles. I had little control over the traffic, but I could choose the route I wanted to drive, the time I left home to head to the university or how I used my time driving – podcasts, thinking and so on.

Example: We all have someone in our professional or personal life that we let 'push our buttons'. I have found that once I identify my reactive behaviour when this happens, the next time I interact with this person, I can take time to think about what my response should be instead of just reacting and saying something that is not productive. I had a faculty member that would often just barge into my office to make a demand for something needed immediately. I remember one of my responses was to yell at her to 'get out of my office right now'. Obviously, that was not a productive interaction. The next time something similar happened, I looked at her, took a deep breath and asked if the issue was urgent or if we could talk once I had completed the task I was involved in at the time. I followed up by going to her office. I sat down and we were able to solve the issue in a short time. She then apologised for the interruption, and we came up with a plan for better resolution of issues. She is to let me know if the matter is urgent, important or both.

HABIT 2 – START WITH THE END IN MIND

Habit 2 is the habit of personal leadership. Covey suggests that one way to think about this habit is to take time to visualise today and then think about the end of your life and how you will be thought of. To begin with the end in mind means starting with a clear understanding of the destination. He tells us that all things are created twice – first mental, then physical. The mental or first creation is based on very clear principles that set the foundation for the physical creation. In other words, it is our blueprint. For the best long-term results, we establish a principle-centred focus for visualisation of the outcomes.

Example: I have found that in working with faculty or students on projects, if I can give them a good idea of the intended results then they can use their time wisely. An example for the faculty is when revising our policy and procedure manual, I took one example and put it in the new format, shared it with them and then distributed certain policies to each person to review. With students, providing them with a good example of a previous paper or project or even the grading rubric lets them focus on a productive outcome.

HABIT 3 – FIRST THINGS FIRST

Habit 3 is the personal fruit of Habits 1 and 2. Habit 3 lets us practise self-management by becoming principle centred and understanding the long-term plan. We focus on time management – the physical creation from Habit 2's mental creation. Covey identifies a strategy for thinking about the best use of our time. He calls it the time management matrix where we compare things that are urgent versus those that are important. (Insert matrix.) Urgent means that an activity requires immediate attention; Importance has to do with the results. Urgent matters lead to reaction. Important matters let us use a proactive approach.

Quadrant I is urgent and important – these are generally considered crises or problems; we all have some of these in our life. Too much time here can lead to stress and burnout, the feeling that we are always putting out fires.

Quadrant II is the heart of effective personal management and includes things that are not urgent but are important. These are the planning and preparation activities that support our success. Results of time in II can lead to control, vision, balance and perspective and fewer crises.

Quadrant III is urgent but not important; activities in this quadrant are deceptive because we are busy and think we are getting real work done but often these are based on the priorities of others. In this quadrant, we have short-term focus and crisis management often with a feeling of no control.

Quadrant IV is the quadrant that is not important and not urgent. It is often where we go to escape the demands of the other quadrants. Too much time here can lead to total irresponsibility, but at times we really do need to take time for ourselves to recharge in Quadrant IV.

Covey suggests that we spend most of our time and effort in Quadrants I and II, realising that we will need to spend time in III and IV at times. The Quadrant II approach lets us say 'no' and focus on 'first things'. Tools that are valuable to move to Quadrant II are those of calendars, planning and identifying priorities.

Example: I managed my calendar online using the Outlook calendar. Activities were colour coded to reflect personal, professional, work, family and so on. I added everything important to my calendar – from my non-routine professional events to our Friday night dinners with friends. Routine and regular meetings were always blocked. I added time for exercise as well as social activities as the 'big' rocks so that I could prioritise deadlines and activities. Quadrant II activities of planning and writing were added as well. Since travel time is important due to traffic where we lived and worked, I tried to add that to the calendar so that anyone who had access to my calendar could determine my availability. I always kept a list to the side of things to do if I had small chunks of time – these were not high-priority or urgent activities but could be considered important. I planned for the week ahead on Friday and for the day by reviewing my calendar at the end of each day.

HABIT 4 – THINK WIN-WIN

Habit 4 is the habit of interpersonal leadership and focuses on the mutual benefit involved. Before we can discuss the dynamics of win-win, let's explore the idea of an emotional bank account. An emotional bank account is like a financial bank account – we make deposits and withdrawals. The deposits in the emotional bank account indicate the amount of trust. The more the trust, the more reserve we have for withdrawals. To understand our relationship with another we must understand what they consider deposits and withdrawals. Covey suggests there are six major deposits we can make – understanding the individual, attending to little things like kindness and courtesies, keeping commitments, clarifying expectations, showing personal integrity and apologising sincerely when you make a withdrawal.

Win-win is not a technique; it is a philosophy of interaction and one of six paradigms – win-win, win-lose, lose-win, lose-lose, win or no deal. The win-win paradigm is the mindset of constantly seeking mutual benefit in all human interactions. It means that we should be open to finding an alternative to a solution that neither party may have thought of – a third alternative.

Example: In trying to give you an example, I realised that I do not now remember a time that this was not my way of thinking – how we can come up with a win-win solution. One of the best examples is when my daughter was just independent in driving and wanted to go out on her own; my husband was not in support, but through thinking win-win we came up with a solution that all three of us agreed would work. There are so many times in my professional life that I have used this approach – sometimes we think of it as brainstorming, but it is so much more than that. It is finding the most important outcome for the parties involved, listening and discussing options that would realise our objectives.

HABIT 5 – SEEK FIRST TO UNDERSTAND, THEN TO BE UNDERSTOOD

Can you remember when you were taught to read and write? I can. But were we ever really taught to listen? Empathic listening is using our eyes, ears and heart to really listen to the other person. It means we give our full attention and allow the other person to have space to talk to us. Empathic listening is an emotional bank account deposit. Covey also uses the analogy of diagnosing before prescribing … trying to understand fully before finding the true issue. Once someone feels understood we open communication and can resolve most issues readily.

Example: I had a staff member who could talk and talk and talk when asking for resolution of an issue. Using my eyes, ears and heart, I would try to focus on his talking so that we could pinpoint the real issue. By doing this, he realised that we had clarified the issue and as that happened, he had identified possible solutions. Once we had those, we could then figure out the best one to apply in this case. He complimented me one time when he said, 'I love talking to you because you "get" me'.

HABIT 6 – SYNERGISE

Habit 6 is based on the principle of creative cooperation. Covey defines synergy when 1 + 1 = more than 2. Synergy can be exciting as we learn to value creativity and celebrate diversity.

Example: I was president of our state professional organisation, and during the first board meeting I was to preside over 17 board members. I thought that the best outcome would be for us to take an issue to discuss and come to a resolution quickly. However, much to my surprise, there was always one person who seemed to be contrary and kept identifying the challenges or views that we had not considered. What I thought should take a few minutes could take an hour. That evening as I processed the meeting, I realised that we made a much better decision because we had heard various sides of the issue. It was my 'Aha!' moment that helped me understand this idea of Habit 6 so much better. Now, when I am putting workgroups together, I seek as much diversity as possible so that we can enrich our discussions and decisions.

HABIT 7 – SHARPEN THE SAW

Habit 7 is the habit of renewal and balance. It allows us to have the capability to use all the other habits – we can be strong in the four dimensions of health – physical, social, spiritual and mental. Sharpening the saw means exercising in all four areas, and to do this we must be proactive. We build these activities into our schedule as Quadrant II activities. We invest in ourselves. Covey uses the analogy of being too busy driving to stop and get gas.

Example: Personally, I had sacrificed some of my regular exercise routines to find time to get more work done. It did not take long to feel worn down and emotionally stressed. Adding back even short outdoor walks on a regular basis started to change both my physical and mental health. We all know that we need to have strength in tough times. To have strength we need to be in our best shape, so it is essential to get exercise, rest and restoration mentally, emotionally and spiritually.

I love to read and the year that I was working on my dissertation, I felt that I would be sacrificing my recreational reading. However, I rewarded myself each day with a 15- to 20-minute reward of pleasure reading after getting work done on my dissertation. It ended up being the case that I read more novels that year than almost any before or after … and I finished my dissertation on time.

Dr. Covey died in 2012, but his family continues his legacy. I would encourage you if interested to read the book in its entirety and perhaps seek out some of the other resources provided by the Franklin Covey organisation. It has made a tremendous difference in my life.

Five Key Takeaways

1. Life/work alignment is a worthy goal that carries many benefits to health, relationships and personal and work satisfaction.
2. The nature of sports physiotherapy means we need to define what life/work alignment means in our context.
3. There are several methods we can apply to help us move towards a feeling of life/work alignment – see above.
4. Alignment will help you feel in tune, synchronised and ready for anything.
5. Find a book that inspires you, a 'quake book' … one that continues to resonate with you over the years.

Five Self-Directed Reflections

1. What does alignment mean to you?
2. Can you nurture more alignment between work and home?
3. How often do you practise self-compassion?
4. Can you identify your boundaries between work and home life?
5. What is a book you would happily reread again and again, and why? What value or joy does it give you?

Reference

Covey, S. (1997). *The 7 habits of highly effective people*. New York, NY: Simon & Schuster.

CHAPTER 13

Dealing With Stress

Derek Lawrance ■ Sergio Martin-Acuna

'Optimism. One of the most important qualities of a good leader is optimism, a pragmatic enthusiasm for what can be achieved. Even in the face of difficult choices and less than ideal outcomes, an optimistic leader does not yield to pessimism. Simply put, people are not motivated or energised by pessimists.'
– Robert Iger, *The Ride of a Lifetime: Lessons Learned from 15 Years as CEO of the Walt Disney Company*

CHAPTER OUTLINE

Introduction

Stress is an inevitable part of life that can have both positive and negative effects on our mental and emotional wellbeing. As children, we may have enjoyed a carefree lifestyle, but as adults, we must learn to manage stressors to prevent depression and anxiety. Managing stress requires effort, patience and practice, as well as the development of healthy coping mechanisms. In this chapter, we will explore the importance of understanding the concept of stress, identifying its causes and developing healthy coping mechanisms to reduce its negative impact on our lives. We have decided to write it in a format that we feel will make it readily accessible and readable. Enjoy.

Preparing My Younger Self for a Better Future

Reflecting on our childhood, we may see a carefree, fun-loving time without any stress. However, for most people, this lifestyle is not sustainable. Life has its ebbs and flows that can affect our perception of stress and carefree living. As adults, it's essential to understand how to manage stressors during our growth phases in life.

If we had the opportunity to teach our younger selves about managing stress, we could start by explaining the concept of stress and how it can be good or bad. It's crucial to understand the difference between the two to make a better decision. Good stressors can come in various forms,

131

such as choosing a favourite snack or purchasing a new car. However, bad stressors require better decision-making abilities and managing them positively can prevent depression and anxiety.

Managing stress is a part of life and we cannot avoid it. Instead, we must identify it and understand the solution to handling it. To manage stress, we need to analyse what's causing it and determine why it's stressing us out. When stressors are out of our control, we need to be flexible and accept that these things can happen. But we have the power to control our emotional response to the stress created. We can calm our nerves or find avenues to release some anger and move on.

When stress is created within our control, we need to accept our decisions and actions that have led to the moment of stress. We cannot rewrite the past, but we can internalise those situations, correct them and identify them in the future. By doing this, we can manage future controllable stressors and ensure positive outcomes.

Learning to manage stress is a continuous process that requires effort, patience and practice. We must develop the habit of self-reflection and learn to prioritise our mental and emotional wellbeing. There are several ways to cope with stress, including exercise, meditation and talking to someone we trust. These practices can help us deal with stress in a healthy way and prevent it from taking over our lives.

By understanding the concept of stress, identifying its causes and developing healthy coping mechanisms, we can reduce its negative impact on our lives. It is never too late to start managing stress positively and by doing so, you can lead a more fulfilling and productive life.

Overcoming Stress and Coping With Adversity

One of the biggest setbacks to managing stress is when it starts to consume your mind and affect your thought processes, leading to feelings of depression and anxiety. Everyone copes with stress differently and it's not always easy to find a solution and act right away. Stress can be overwhelming, persistent and even debilitating at times, affecting our nerves and weighing us down. However, with experience and resilience, we can learn to cope with it more effectively.

Allowing stress to take a toll on our bodies and mental wellbeing can be damaging and demoralising. It's important to recognise the signs and signals of this, and education on managing stress should be a priority during our childhood and adolescent years. As we age, we experience various life events that can cause stress, such as work-related stress, relationship stress, financial stress and health-related stress. It's pivotal to have a solid understanding of how to manage these stressors to ensure that we don't fall into a cycle of depression and anxiety.

Mental health awareness has seen a significant increase in recent years, with more people realising the impact that stress can have on one's mental health, potentially leading to other issues. Equipping ourselves with proper skill sets and tools can help us avoid the debilitating effects of stress.

Lessons From Success

I have been fortunate to have amazing mentors that taught me the importance of celebrating both successes and failures in life, as they are both a great opportunity to become a better healthcare provider and grow as a student and early professional. My biggest mentor? My father. Since I started playing sports, he would always talk about the importance of prioritising the journey and embracing the process more than the wins or the losses. Nowadays, as an early professional athletic trainer working in the professional setting, I try to keep his wise words very present by embracing the journey and celebrating every small success. This profession requires us to be efficient in high-pressure situations and sometimes that might blind us from enjoying how privileged we are to be doing what we love. Every success must be celebrated.

Our job involves dealing with the lowest point of our patient population since injuries directly affect the level of performance, and consequently playing time. That's when the role of the Sports Medicine Team becomes the most important, since we not only must rehab the patient, but we must also provide the right environment for the patient to always feel physically and psychologically motivated to approach a rehab that might last weeks, months or years. In these situations, it is essential to show and educate the athletes on the importance of learning how to celebrate every small success through goal setting – short-, mid- and long-term goals. For example, I have experienced cases in which having an athlete with an anterior cruciate ligament reconstruction score baseline or minimal deficit numbers in a maximal voluntary isometric contraction strength test is celebrated as much as a goal in the extra time, a buzzer-beater, a hole in one or a pole position.

Learning to celebrate small successes and acknowledge their importance in the entire journey is essential but is not easy to do. During my senior year in college, I was the Chair of the Outreach Subcommittee and District 1 Representative of the National Athletic Trainers' Association (NATA) Student Leadership Committee, President of the Athletic Training Student Association at my University and Member of the Student Leadership Committee and Young Professional Committee workgroup. While doing that, I was an athletic training seasonal intern for a Major League Soccer team, studying for the Board of Certification Exam, and job hunting for an athletic training graduate assistantship position. In addition to all my responsibilities, the world was involved in one of the biggest health crises of the decade due to the COVID-19 pandemic. Listening to and taking advice from my mentors, Michael Goldenberg and Dr. Jeff Konin, was important, as I was dealing with a very stressful time in my life, and they both helped and educated me on managing the anxiety I was experiencing due to the uncertainty, as well as to embrace and enjoy the process as unique as it was. Due to the lack of job positions, I started experiencing some stress associated with potentially not landing my desired position, which could potentially affect my visa status in the country. Mike and Jeff made sure I was doing okay, and not only did they help me with my responsibilities in the NATA committees, but they also used their extensive network to help me land a graduate assistantship job at a great institution.

To recap, enjoy the journey and always celebrate success, but make sure to celebrate failure as well and approach it as a growth opportunity with positivity and optimism. Failure is part of life, and instead of letting it cause stress, we should be thankful for the opportunity of being able to do what we love.

Balancing Wellbeing With Ambition

When you progress in your career, you tend to focus on the bigger picture, which is professional development and personal growth. These two ideas go hand in hand as we mature and find ourselves excelling in our career paths. However, it doesn't always come easy, and it doesn't always move along as smoothly as you would think.

Early on in my life and career I knew generally where I wanted to be and how my personal life would look. I would work towards excelling as an athletic trainer and eventually develop into a leader. Personally, I know I wanted to have a family. When these two paths merged into one, stressful situations were more persistent than ever. Why, though? You'd think that progressing in a career you love with a family you love even more would allow you to have endless happiness. What you don't see is how people find ways to balance each aspect of their life, in unison.

At one point, I faced a significant peak in my stress levels. I had uprooted my life to chase a dream job across the country and, years later, found myself as a Director of Health and Performance for a professional soccer team. While I thought I had everything I wanted, I realised I could push myself further by going back to school to earn my doctorate degree. However, I didn't anticipate the added complexity of becoming a father and supporting our newly expanded family.

By the end of 2021, I was managing a performance department with a professional soccer team, working on my doctorate and managing a home life that now included being a dad and supporting my recovering wife. This went on for a few months and I felt as though I was handling it well, but I started to get a sense that it might be overwhelming. I found myself in the evenings staring at a computer screen after having spent 10 hours at work, 4 hours at home cleaning, feeding, cooking and now facing 2 to 3 hours of homework. Stress levels were getting maxed out.

The stress became overwhelming as I tried to balance my work, studies, home life and a new role as a dad. It felt like there weren't enough hours in the day. To make matters worse, my wife and I decided to leave our jobs and move closer to our family to provide the best care for our daughter. Suddenly, I was unemployed, studying for my doctorate and facing the daunting task of finding new work in a new area.

Countless days going into it all, I had self-reflections thinking, 'How am I going to be the best dad possible, a supporting husband and a student, and find a way to make money to support all of the above?' I decided to do what any sane person would do, and I started reaching out to peers. I needed to speak to people who have been through a change of jobs or locations and, most importantly, balancing all that with families.

In those moments of stress, I found it helpful to focus on the following to help me tackle my challenges and find balance:

1. Breathe – take moments to appreciate where you are and find ways or exercises to get your mind off what is stressing you out.
2. Focus on the positives – looking at all the good that has come from personal care and preparation to feel comfortable in an uncomfortable situation.
3. Speak to peers – asking for advice and help lends itself to understanding how others may have been through similar situations.
4. Create a plan – doing nothing is the worst thing you can do. Find realistic opportunities to support your goals.

It's essential to remember that solutions exist even in the most difficult situations. It's crucial to take a step back, reflect and develop a step-by-step process to create balance and peace of mind. By implementing these strategies, I was able to overcome my stress and find success in both my personal and professional life.

Prevention Is Key

Athletic training and sports medicine is a profession in which stress is present and sometimes not easy to manage – think about prevention, like preventing injuries. We must respond to highly stressful situations, like dealing with life-threatening cases or making decisions under pressure that involve the athletes, coaches, stakeholders and more. Therefore, it is important to stay up to date and educated on proper stress management as well as to learn to identify the stressors and potential signs of burnout so that it can be properly dealt with. This is a big topic nowadays in the industry, and NATA is advocating for educating and providing resources to ensure these issues are being identified, with the purpose of coming up with the necessary measures to solve and mitigate them to achieve a proper work-life balance and be effective and efficient.

The first step is to identify stress and burnout. One of the initial signs is a decreased level of emotional readiness and desire to continue working. The best way to identify it is by acknowledging a lack of motivation and emotional detachment from co-workers, patients and cases. In these situations, it is essential to take a step back and analyse the 'Why' and potential causes. We tend to neglect ourselves when we experience stress, and talking with somebody from our support system is the best route to identify and acknowledge the stressor in order to learn how to react in a positive way. Whether it is a family member, a mentor, a friend or a professional, the identification and outcome will be better if you express your feelings and rely on somebody. Not only will you feel supported, but most importantly, by listening to somebody's unbiased feedback, you will have a different perspective that will help you better understand and manage the stress. Take a step back, analyse the situation and take some time to decompress and refocus.

The second step is creating a routine. As a young professional, the routine that I was able to develop after talking with multiple mentors and reading some articles from Timothy Neal included taking more active control of my sleeping habits, nutrition and hydration, as well as exercising every day twice (one of them being outdoors). In addition, I realised that investing more time in my family and loved ones, together with performing daily mindfulness through fire meditation, helped me get back on track and take control of my stress and work-life balance.

Do not forget to take care of yourself, establish boundaries and maintain work-life balance. That will allow you to enjoy your job, and as Mark Twain used to say, 'you will never have to work a day in your life'.

Advice for Someone Starting Their Career

Entering the profession of athletic training involves a stressful transition. A certified athletic trainer must go through at least 6 years of education and clinical preparation in order to be eligible for the board of certification exam. Once the exam is passed and both the certification and the licensure are approved, early professionals need to establish the foundation of their career, which in the healthcare profession often means working in roles that involve a poor work-life balance and low financial compensation. Athletic trainers have an essential role in any setting, but a lot of early professionals find themselves experiencing early burnout and leaving the profession because they are trying to deal with the poor conditions that are part of that initial phase of their careers.

On the other hand, if there is a time to 'put in the work', it is as an early professional, with the main goals of gaining experience, growing as a provider and establishing interprofessional relationships. A good piece of advice that I took from peers and mentors is that as a student and early professional, it is important to start setting a foundation of good habits and hard work, but boundaries need to be established and a proper work-life balance is being set. Working hard is important, but learning how to manage stress early on is essential to avoid burnout and stay efficient and motivated. Make sure to spend time with family and loved ones, try to exercise at least 30 minutes a day, spend time outdoors and try to perform some mindfulness or meditation while having some alone time. At the age of 27, and with 3 years of experience at the professional level, those are the habits that I have established in order to maintain a proper work-life balance.

Managing stress as a student and early professional athletic trainer is not easy, and as of today, even with the current knowledge I have, it is still a challenge. Investing time and staying involved with your university, local, state and national associations is helpful to learn how to cope with stressors. By staying active and volunteering in committees and workgroups, you will be able to network with amazing professionals that will become your mentors and will guide you through the rest of your career. When I was a junior in college, while attending the Eastern Athletic Trainers Association Annual Conference in Boston, I had the privilege of meeting a great friend and mentor, Michael Goldenberg. Michael, also 'Mike' for friends and colleagues, is a legend of the profession and one of the biggest leaders in the NATA, as well as a member of the Hall of Fame. His work has helped immensely advance the profession, and on a personal level he has helped me grow as a leader and create good habits to manage stress while staying productive. Since then, I have relied on him, along with my good friend Dr. Jeff Konin, for every important decision that I have had to take regarding my career as an athletic trainer.

The main takeaway is that stress will always be present in your life, and that is inevitable. How to identify the stressors and manage them is the key. Relying on people that have been through the same situations and come out successfully is essential to take the necessary steps to ensure you are successful as well. Stay involved and connect with mentorship programs – having mentors will change your professional and personal life.

Looking Back as if You Were 80 Years Old

Stress management is vital to be successful at any job and proper management is essential for a good work-life balance. Athletic training and sports medicine providers are exposed to highly stressful situations, including life-threatening conditions. Therefore, it is important to manage the work-life balance and outside stressors that can affect mental health so that the work performed in those high-pressure situations can be sharp and efficient.

I was extremely fortunate to have a support system that helped me in moments of my career when I struggled handling stress and work-life balance, which consequently affected my mental and physical health. After talking with the sports psychologist at the university I was attending, I was able to identify the stressors that were affecting my health, starting with my nutritional habits. I realised that because of the amount of time that I was spending working and studying, I started skipping meals and having a low and unhealthy calorie intake. Instead of eating regular meals, I was fasting during the day and eating only unhealthy and fast food late at night. In addition, I was not exercising and barely spending any time outdoors outside of work, which consequently developed into poor sleeping habits that affected my energy levels and overall mood. This cycle went on for months until I decided to seek advice, which then helped me identify the stressors and take a step back to analyse each one and take action to change. During the process, I learned about the changes of stage from various models, and it slowly helped to start planning and acting on my stress management.

It took me around 6 months to get adjusted and stick to the routine but being able to find a healthy balance in stress management was the best advice I have ever had, and since then I have been able to approach every day with a positive mindset and good energy. We deal with stress daily, but it doesn't always have to be a negative approach, as it allows us to stay motivated to achieve tasks and goals. When we let stress take over our life, that is when it can start affecting both our mental and physical health, and that is the moment to seek help and guidance.

Stress is inevitable, so do not be afraid to ask and be vocal if things don't go well. Trying to solve it by yourself will never be as successful as relying on people that have dealt with the same issue in a successful manner. Remember that stress is a positive thing if you keep it well balanced, as it will help you to stay productive and achieve goals, which will lead to personal and professional growth.

Something Else to Consider

It is a widely held belief that most people wish they had the skills to manage stress without having to endure difficult situations in life. Coping with stress can be one of the most challenging aspects of anyone's life, and as we all know, stress can strike at any time, at any place and under any circumstances. This is what makes it such a difficult challenge to deal with.

However, as we gain experience with age, we can reflect on our past experiences and use them as a guide to help us navigate future stressful situations. But just imagine if we had been given the tools and knowledge to handle such situations before they even occurred. This is an idea that many of us can relate to in some way. Unfortunately, life is not always that simple and we often must learn important lessons the hard way.

Experience can teach us many valuable lessons, both good and bad, but the key is to always find a way to apply the knowledge gained from those experiences. One of the most common questions we ask ourselves is, 'How do we apply what we have learned when we have a new challenge?'

Sometimes we don't have all the answers, but we can always seek guidance from our past experiences. This is the foundation of our ability to adapt to stress. Think about all the times this has happened to you – a new job, a new city, meeting new people, social gatherings and so on. Each new situation presents its own unique challenges and stressors, but we have the ability, thanks to our experiences and learned coping mechanisms, to apply the strategies that work best for us.

Five Key Takeaways

1. Managing stress is a part of life that cannot be avoided. It is essential to identify the causes of stress and seek solutions to handle it, bearing in mind that there is good stress, known as eustress, and bad stress, or distress.
2. Coping with stress is a continuous process that requires effort, patience and practice.
3. Equipping ourselves with proper skill sets and tools can help us avoid the debilitating effects of stress.
4. Celebrating both successes and failures in life is essential to becoming a better healthcare provider and human being.
5. It is important to recognise the signs and signals of stress and prioritise education on how to manage it during childhood and adolescence.

Five Self-Directed Reflections

1. Identify the stressors in your life – can you eliminate some of them?
2. Do you have a toolkit to use when under stress?
3. How often do you consider the balance of work, and the stress that accompanies it, with your wellbeing?
4. Think about when you face a challenge or point of adversity. How do you usually respond? Could you respond differently?
5. Do you have a practice to build up exposure to small bouts of stress to improve your capacity, as a small prevention tool?

Journeys

Setbacks, Success, Personal Stories and Reflections – Wayne Diesel

Introduction: 'My Long Walk to Retirement'

My professional career as a physiotherapist spanned over 30 years, across three continents and multiple elite sporting organisations. The lessons learnt, I believe, have led to tremendous personal growth and a greater appreciation of the many life-changing opportunities available to those who are prepared to challenge themselves. My latest challenge is working as a performance consultant with a truly inspirational group of Red Bull's downhill mountain bike riders based in North Wales. The aim of this chapter is to share some of these lessons and personal experiences.

The title of my journey, 'My long walk to retirement', is a tribute to Nelson Mandela's autobiography *The Long Walk to Freedom*. Whilst I fully accept that my long walk in no way compares to Mandela's long walk, it was his story and leadership that provided much of my inspiration to overcome challenges, use lessons learnt, embrace differences and acknowledge the sacrifices made by our loved ones. It was during my time as part of the South African rugby management team that I personally witnessed the amazing leadership skills of Nelson Mandela.

This chapter will highlight many of the lessons I learnt, inside and outside the realm of sport, that helped shape my professional career. By sharing these lessons, I hope to inspire others to pursue their dreams, believe in themselves and complete the cycle by mentoring the next generation.

Uncovering a Passion

A couple of years prior to graduating as a physiotherapist in 1987, from the University of Witwatersrand in South Africa, I had a motorbike accident. This accident, which caused a thoracic vertebral wedge compression fracture, meant that I was no longer able to represent my university in the upcoming South African universities soccer tournament. Having just been selected to play, I was asked by our team's management if I would instead be interested in providing physiotherapy for the team during the tournament. Accepting this opportunity, I discovered a passion for working in sport, which would propel me to work with teams across the world.

Over the next 30-plus years, I was fortunate to have worked in seven different major sports across three continents. Arguably, an even bigger positive outcome of this adversity was meeting my future wife, Jean.

The Importance of Resilience

Resilience is a life skill that evolves from learning to cope with adversity. Coaches worldwide recognise resilience as an extremely valuable attribute of their players. Over the years it became apparent to me that players who returned to play after a significant injury appeared to display more resilience than players who never had to deal with a severe injury, and I suggested as much to Mike Tannenbaum, then president of football operations of the Miami Dolphins during my first NFL Combine.

Empowered Leadership

I have on multiple occasions witnessed the impact that leadership has on a team's performance. An example of strong leadership was during my time with Gloucester Rugby. Our head coach, Nigel Melville, actively empowered players to lead by allowing them to influence tactics for upcoming games. In the week leading up to a game, players from each position would present their thoughts on how best to deal with the opposition's strengths and weaknesses. By analysing their opponent and presenting their findings, the players were better prepared for the game. The effect that this had on decision-making and successful outcomes during games was profound. During halftime, players would again be involved in discussing any changes in the opponents' strategy and how best to deal with them. Contrary to this, I have witnessed situations where players are simply told by the coaches what to do, with little or no buy-in of the strategy. In these situations, the players either did not fully understand their roles or were too slow to react when opponents suddenly changed strategy, increasing the likelihood of losing.

Leaders who empower others, such as teammates or colleagues, to lead increase their chances of success. This is especially relevant in the interdisciplinary performance team environment where the head of the department cannot be highly skilled in all services provided to the team. My approach was therefore to allow the doctors, strength and conditioning coaches, sports scientists, physiotherapists, athletic trainers, psychologists, nutritionists and other specialists to lead in their area of expertise and to collaborate. My role was to help coordinate and focus interactions between the specialties so that we could have 'one voice' when it came to communicating with the player, coaches, owner and other administrative staff.

Being Accountable to All

The value closely related to leadership is accountability. Players holding other players accountable for their performances appeared to have a significantly greater impact than a member of the coaching staff pointing out a player's errors. The 2013 Carling Cup Final, where Tottenham Hotspur beat Chelsea to win the cup, highlighted what accountability meant to performance and helped shape my management style. Because my staff and I were seen as being collectively responsible for the service we provided, accountability was encouraged.

Providing medical care for players demands preparation and attention to detail. The level of preparation should never be underestimated, and medical emergencies can and do happen when least expected. I have also witnessed how some of the very best athletes and coaches, regardless of their sport, leave no stone unturned in preparing. This detailed preparation is often confused with superstition, where top athletes have a set routine before games. Setting specific routines helps players to prepare and therefore perform consistently at their best.

Teamwork

Teamwork is another value I've developed throughout my career. Whilst this chapter will not discuss everything that goes into creating positive teamwork, it will discuss the value of teamwork. All team sports actively encourage teamwork and go about team building in many ways. Failure to carry out or recognise an opponent's play can result in a bad play or even injury. Being prepared to put your body on the line to protect a teammate, even at the risk of severe injury, involves the highest level of teamwork that I have witnessed in sport.

Being Scientific About Life

It is imperative to examine life's data, just as one would do for academic data. I began to recognise the negative impact that Apartheid had on me. I learnt, through sport, in particular working with Bafana Bafana (South African soccer team) during the African Cup of Nations in 1998, to embrace and respect cultural differences, and it was during that tournament I finally felt relaxed when working with players and staff of different ethnicities. I have learnt the value of communicating when the perspective of someone else does not match my own, and in trying to understand their perspective. Sport has been widely recognised as playing a major role in bringing South Africans of all cultures together.

Once I left South Africa, I was again fortunate enough to work with teams where cultural differences were welcomed and viewed as adding to a team's strength. The other important lesson that I learnt regarding diversity was that players from different countries and cultures had varied expectations and preferences regarding medical treatment types. Using a one-size-fits-all treatment approach may limit the perceived efficacy and buy-in from players. My personal experiences regarding the importance of embracing diverse treatment methods or beliefs have included a range of traditional healers.

When I was in private practice in South Africa, I was seeing an elite long-distance runner for an Achilles problem. He was improving slowly and then suddenly stopped seeing me. After several weeks he came back into the clinic and told me he was feeling much better. I assumed that he had followed my advice on eccentric exercises but was intrigued when he showed me several lacerations along the Achilles tendon. It turns out that he had been to see a traditional healer who used a razor blade to make small incisions to 'expel the evil spirits'.

Another case involved a professional rugby player that I had seen with a torn posterior cruciate ligament (PCL). The orthopaedic surgeon recommended surgery, but the player was reluctant. Instead, he visited a faith healer, T. B. Joshua, from Nigeria. On return the surgeon re-examined the knee and found it to be stable and said he could return to rugby. This case highlighted the power of faith, as he was a devout Christian. The take-home lesson from all of this was that players need to trust and believe in you and the proposed treatment plan.

Learning and Autonomy

Autonomy is a key factor in providing quality medical care that will ensure trust. A cornerstone of autonomy is informed consent, and informed consent requires player education. The lesson here is that we as practitioners have a moral duty and obligation to keep abreast of current evidence-based medical practice. This is one of the biggest challenges facing medical staff because of the ever-changing scientific landscape and technological advancements.

I have always enjoyed learning and found out that teaching was one of the best ways for me to learn. Hence, after obtaining my physiotherapy degree in 1986 I went on to receive a BSc (Med) (Hons) in Sport Science in 1988 and ultimately a PhD in 1994. Today I remain academically involved through reviewing scientific articles, lecturing, presenting and joining a scientific advisory board. This passion for learning, I believe, has provided me with a range of skills and often an appreciation of skills that other therapists can provide. Getting players to feel comfortable deciding, in an informed manner, upon treatment options is becoming the norm in high-performance teams today.

Focusing on the Person, Not the Injury

Returning to play following a traumatic injury has not only physical implications for the player but often psychological ones too. Biopsychosocial models are currently being used in return-to-play programmes by high-performance departments. Education, as described earlier, has proved successful in reducing the injured players' levels of stress and anxiety. The four pillars of the programme are engagement, empowering, feedback and transparency. Engagement involves player education and consultation, which empowers the player to contribute their thoughts on treatment or exercise options. Rehab 'vacations' at appropriate stages of the programme include input from the player. Feedback includes regular video footage of their movement patterns to highlight progress or areas that require improvement. Regular meetings with the player, performance staff, coaches and front office executives create transparency in the programme. This player-centred approach also strongly encourages personal and professional development during the rehab phase. Once when working with a player who had successfully returned to his sport, he stated how confident he had been in the process and coped better mentally because he understood and felt involved throughout. Months later the coaches also commented on how much his shooting and leadership skills had improved. The valuable lesson I learnt from this process was the importance of meaningful involvement of players in decision-making for their health and performance.

Last, but Not Least

The final lesson I would like to discuss is the importance of family. My family have collectively and individually made tremendous sacrifices for me to work across the globe. The support given by my family has made this journey not only possible but also extremely rewarding. Almost every team that I have worked for has attempted to promote the feeling of being a 'family'. In cases where players, as well as staff, have felt a strong family bonds, the performance remained at consistently high levels and a happier mood prevailed. This does not mean that there were no disagreements. Instead, everyone felt comfortable raising concerns and that their opinion mattered.

This long walk to retirement has been extremely fulfilling, and I want to thank the hundreds of athletes, coaches, support staff and my family for teaching me so many valuable lessons. So, on reflection, my message to anyone reading this is to follow your dreams and be prepared to continue learning.

Setbacks, Success, Personal Stories and Reflections – Ian Horsley

Introduction

It was never in my life plan to become a physiotherapist. I always thought that I wanted to be a surgeon.

I can't remember what it was that made me want to be a surgeon. And I don't even remember deciding what type of surgeon I wanted to be. But for as long as I can remember when anyone asked me, 'What do you want to be when you go up?' I used to say, 'I would like to be a surgeon'.

The Journey Starts With a Single Step

With that in mind, I joined St John's Ambulance Brigade and learned some basic first aid skills (I thought it would look good on my university application and give me a rudimentary understanding of injury management) whilst I was at school. I diligently worked through my (as they were then) 'O' levels to attain the number of grades that I needed to be able to go on then to Sixth Form College and do the required 'A' levels in order to get into medical school.

So, when I got to Sixth Form College, having been hard working when I was at school, I got distracted a little bit more by sport. I was always interested in sport and played an awful lot of sport, but I was probably more interested in girls, and my focus on my work drifted a little bit. Needless to say, when my 'A' level results came out for physics, chemistry, biology, sports studies and general studies, I had not made the grade to get into medical school. Suddenly my life plan was becoming derailed!

Around the same time that this happened the Miners' Strike started (6 March 1984 to 3 March 1985). I live in a mining community in Yorkshire, and at that time both my parents were employed by (what was then) the National Coal Board; both my parents were on strike for a year, and therefore we weren't getting any income into the house. I stayed back at Sixth Form College and repeated a few of my 'A' levels and helped support the family any way I could during the miners' strike. When I repeated my 'A' levels my results were better but not good enough to get into any medical school on a second attempt. Time for a rethink.

The Plan in Liverpool

But I was offered a place at Liverpool University studying physiology, which had a common first year with medicine. And there was some talk that if you performed well enough in your exams at the end of year one, there would be a possibility that you might get accepted for medicine in your second year. This was my plan.

I settled into Liverpool University and then in my second term whilst playing rugby league for the university, a significant life event happened that changed the course of my career. Some people might call it a 'lucky break' – I broke my back. I fractured my lumbar spine, playing rugby league. And whilst being managed through the 3 months which necessitated me being encased in a full thoracic plaster cast that was renewed every couple of weeks, during this time, I watched what happened from my care and sort of realised that the doctors in the medical profession that I came across didn't actually treat me; they organised my treatment and really, at the end, it was the physiotherapist who helped me recover from my problem.

Serendipity

Now again, this is where there seems to be a lot of serendipity in my career, because at that time, one of the guys that I lived in halls with had a girlfriend who was at Withington Hospital School of Physiotherapy, and she was in her first year of study. And I got talking to her and I thought, oh, you know what, that might be a profession for me.

Since I had almost missed a full term due to my injury, I realised that I would not be outstanding in the final exams and ought to have a plan C. I applied to university for the next year to study physiotherapy; however, since I was late applying I didn't get a place, but I was put into clearing and was lucky enough to be given an interview at Withington Hospital School of Physiotherapy in Manchester! Now again, there is a common thread here because whilst I was a physiology student at Liverpool University, they were carrying out some research looking at eutrophic stimulators, which were later to be used for the treatment of Bell's palsy. And I was a guinea pig for one of these units. When I went for my interview at Withington, I discovered that this was the place where the clinical trials were going to be, so again there seemed to be a link there. And after my interview I was awarded a place to study physiotherapy in September 1986.

When I was in my first year at Withington, I came across an article in a journal which was then for the Association of Chartered Physios in Sports Medicine (ACPSM). It was an editorial that said, with the Olympic Games being the highlight of most athletes' career, therefore, sports physios ought to consider that aim for the pinnacle of their career. Now, up until this point, I had not really decided where I wanted to work in physiotherapy, but I thought yeah, that seems like a good pathway. At that time, I had no idea how I was going to follow it – but at least I had a goal!

In my second year of study whilst on clinical placement, within the gym and rehab setting, a local senior rugby club came to the hospital and said, 'We would like a physio for our club. And we'd like somebody who knows something about rugby. So could you let us have somebody?' At that time, I was still playing rugby at Manchester Metropolitan University, and I was doing well on my placement there. My supervisors knew that I played rugby league (since I kept turning up with cuts and bruises), but what they didn't know was that this was a Rugby Union club that was looking for a physiotherapist. Anyway, they suggested that I ought to go down. I duly went down to this rugby club (Brighton Park) and began being a physio with nobody else there – no doctor, no other medical person there. Literally with a bucket and a sponge and the ignorance of youth! This was my introduction to 'sports physiotherapy', and it gave me a great grounding, making me rapidly upskill my knowledge, exposing me to a relatively high level of sport and making links and forging relationships with the medical profession within Manchester. Based on my work with Broughton Park rugby club, I was offered a few positions in private practice when I qualified (in 1989), which I ultimately didn't take up, initially because I wanted to go to the NHS and continue my training. I took a position at Whiston and St. Helens Hospital and started my rotations initially on the elderly care rotation, which I was on there for over 6 months.

Vision, and What's Next?

At the time of my interview for my first post, I was asked the question, 'Where would you like to be with your career in 10 years?' My answer to that question was, 'I'd like to be an England Rugby (Union) physiotherapist' … and so began my new journey!

I got a phone call in the New Year from a physiotherapist who had a private clinic in Manchester who had just been given the job of being England cricket physio and needed someone to cover his practice whilst he was away on tour with the team. Again, this offer came off the back of my elective placement that I did in Rochdale (in my final year of study) with a very renowned physio called Dennis Wright, who had been asked who he would recommend.

My choice to do my elective placement at Rochdale (20 minutes down the road from where I was studying), rather than go somewhere 'exciting' like London or America, was greeted with a few raised eyebrows by my student friends. But Dennis Wright had a great reputation as a sports physiotherapist who had 'been there and done that', and he was a mine of information about management of musculoskeletal injuries.

Varied Experiences

Anyway, after a little bit of soul searching, I thought, well, why not? I went to work in private practice in Manchester. During this time, I was still working with Broughton Park rugby club and I also ended up being the physiotherapist for the England Amputee Football team who were based and trained locally and ended up supporting the team at two football World Cups. (one in Seattle and one in the Soviet Union). Again, valuable experience in travelling with a team on a shoestring budget in sport.

When my time came to an end in Manchester, one of the players who was a junior international Rugby Union player came to see me and I said I was going to move back to Yorkshire to take a position at a clinic in Wakefield (the clinic I now actually own). He said, oh that's good, because he was playing for what was then probably Yorkshire's premier Rugby Union Club, Wakefield FC, and they were looking for a new physio. Again, seems like a little bit of luck on my part. I went down, had an interview and was given the job of physio at Wakefield Rugby Union Club.

The Oval Ball

At this time in what was the amateur era of Rugby Union, the England Rugby Union setup, we used to have the Divisional Championship, where the country was split into four geographical areas, each represented by a team of players associated with each respective area. A championship was played (each team played each other team) and the winner was crowned Divisional Champion. This system helps expose top-level players for England selection. At this time the North of England used Wakefield as a training base. And one night when the North Division were training, their physio wasn't available and they asked me to step in. I stepped in and was asked to continue as North Division physio for the next season.

The doctor who worked with me for England North then went on to become an England Rugby Union senior first-team doctor and rang me the next season to say there was a position available with England Students and he recommended me for that position, which I accepted. I worked with England Students for 4 years and that began my path in sport and in rugby. I worked my way through various teams within the Rugby Football Union (RFU); I worked with England sevens, and I spent most of my career working with the RFU with the England 'A', or England Saxons, as they are also known. I was lucky to work with the elite playing squad in the run-up to the World Cup in 2003, which England ultimately won! So, in a roundabout way I achieved my career goal expressed at my initial interview.

The Olympic Plan

I still had the desire to go to an Olympic Games with Team GB, and I applied for a position for the 2008 Olympic Games but was told I didn't have a wide enough experience of different sports and attendance at a multisport event. Therefore, I needed a new plan.

I saw a job advertised at the English Institute of Sport (the organisation which supports most of the Olympic and Paralympic sports), applied and began working initially 18 hours a week. This exposed me to many different sports, delivering physiotherapy, which put me in a good position for selection to Team England for the 2010 Commonwealth Games, which were to be held in Delhi, India.

The year 2012 was to be the year of the Olympics in London. I applied to be a member of the Team GB medical support team within the headquarters in London. Once again, I was lucky to be selected. I achieved the second goal of my career. My first initial goal was to work with England Rugby and now I have been part of Team GB at an Olympic Games.

I continued my split-role work in private practice and working with the English Institute of Sport. I have been fortunate to be selected for a second Commonwealth Games in 2014 in Edinburgh, the 2016 Olympic Games in Rio and the 2020 Olympics in Tokyo (which ultimately took place in 2021).

The Change Makers

When I look back on my life and I look back on my career, it seems there's been a lot of good luck and good fortune. But I think it's a case of having a vision and sticking to my goals of selecting the right opportunities that would push me towards making the right career decisions.

How Did This Happen?

So here I am, 30-odd years qualified with a successful musculoskeletal practice in Wakefield, West Yorkshire, a Senior Physiotherapist for the English Institute of Sport, a nationally recognised upper limb and shoulder rehab specialist with a PhD. And I think that it's because I kept my 'eyes on the prize'.

Advice

My advice to budding physiotherapists would be …
1. Have a goal, and make that goal as specific as possible (such as England Women's Senior Football Physiotherapist).
2. Give yourself a realistic time frame to complete this goal and factor in other nonprofessional aspirations, such as getting married, having children and developing a social network.
3. Make time to gain experience. There are always opportunities to shadow professional people. It will expose you to the actual makeup of the job – the good and the bad. Experience working with lots of different people and review their 'good' and 'bad' practices; commit to mirroring the 'good' bits and ensuring you don't repeat their 'bad' bits.

4. Finally, be ready for failure – such as failing to get the job you were interviewed for. We all experience failure in our lives, but these are (possibly) the most valuable lessons, especially if we reflect on the feedback given at the time.

The Best Decision

But most importantly, the best decision that I made in my life was marrying my wife, Lynne. She allowed me to pursue my rugby dream, which meant lots of time being away from home when we had two children under the age of 2, and she has enabled me to have a successful practice of which she is the Practice Manager. I couldn't have had the life and career that I had without her love and support and the acceptance from my children – that being away was partly necessary to give them the quality of life which they were used to.

Setbacks, Success, Personal Stories and Reflections – Ritchie Barber

Introduction

I am a physiotherapist with cerebral palsy (CP). My love for physiotherapy first started as I tried to navigate the challenges of living with CP with the support of a physiotherapy team. My admiration was strengthened further throughout my career as a Paralympic swimmer, during which time I won multiple world and European medals and eventually won a silver medal at the Sydney Paralympics in 2000. My biggest career goal was to become the physiotherapist for the British Paralympic swimming team, and after my retirement from swimming and a stint in the National Health Service (NHS), I achieved this, joining the team in 2014. I have also helped Swim England equal their greatest-ever medal haul at the Commonwealth Games 2022 in Birmingham. Alongside my activities in sport, I work for Worsley Physiotherapy and Sports Injury Clinic, a private practice based in Salford, England, and I have taken up a post at the University of Salford to lecture on the BSc (Hons) physiotherapy programme.

My Purpose

Everybody has a purpose in life. I was one of two babies born to my mother the same day. My twin brother was stillborn; delivered first, he ultimately set off a chain of events that led to me suffering a hypoxic brain injury during delivery. This resulted in a permanent physical disability known as cerebral palsy (CP).

My son now carries the same name as my brother.

I sometimes feel I'm moving through life for both of us, and as such I feel a strong sense of accountability to my brother to make sure I don't waste my life, a life that he could have been either experiencing with me or instead of me. So, in essence, my success is his.

About Me

I have been a physiotherapist since 2006. I spent the first 8 years of my career completing my core rotations in hospital settings in the NHS. In 2014 I took the role of lead physiotherapist for British Paralympic swimming, and in 2016 I added athlete health lead for British Paralympic swimming to my title. After 8 years I returned to Salford University, this time to lecture on their BSc (Hons) Physiotherapy programme. Between 1998 and 2004 I swam for the British Paralympic swimming team, winning multiple medals at world and European championships, culminating with a silver medal at the Paralympics in Sydney 2000. My experiences growing up with a disability and my experiences in sport have driven my interest in physiotherapy. My purpose has strengthened my commitment.

Identity

I will not continually introduce myself as being disabled, nor do I expect anyone else in the disabled community to do the same. I freely admit my attitude towards disability may be different than the person next to me who may or may not be disabled. I also admit that I'm privileged when it comes to disability; my impairments are dwarfed by those of many of my friends and the wider disabled community, and, just to be clear, I identify as being disabled but my disability does not define me – that's a path to disablement and reliance on others.

I define my abilities and my scope of practice and see my environment as the limiting factor. I challenge those who can't see this; we should expect this attitude across all facets of physiotherapy and healthcare. I've been under the supervision of people who have focused too much on what my disability might prevent me from doing, rather than on how the environment might limit me. My skills and abilities, irrespective of my disability, are a result of many other people's time and effort; they have all contributed to my identity as a physiotherapist. I'm defined by their combined efforts. How does that improve me as a physiotherapist?

They all created a better me, as a person and physiotherapist.

Greatest Achievements

My greatest achievement is becoming a physiotherapist; second, winning my silver medal at the Sydney 2000 Paralympic games, and I suppose rightly so.

Some of my darkest days were during high school, where I was the only physically disabled student. To make matters worse, all my friends from primary school went to a different high school, so I was alone in a new environment, starting on the back foot in so many ways. I was bullied for 4 years straight – physically, psychologically and socially. I was isolated, and initially I suffered in silence. Eventually, two important things happened. First, I found education, and second, I found a voice. The former was driven mainly by the need to find a level playing field and the latter was eventually driven by sheer desperation.

Studying became my superstrength. I felt the only way to get out of this 'hell hole' was to study hard and study fast. I eventually left high school with nine good general certificates of secondary education (GCSEs), and more importantly I'd earned the right to study A-levels at college. I remember the day I told my parents about the bullying; they were devastated. But by speaking up and finding my voice, I found the motivation to succeed in this environment, especially when they suggested I move schools. This suggestion seemed to give me greater robustness and resilience to fight on. When I look back on this period of my life, it is clear that with each passing year two things grew: my sense of achievement and my gratitude to the bullies who have contributed in a strangely positive way to where I am today and, more importantly, who I am.

Being a recipient of the Mussabini Medal, a sports award recognising the coaches of British sports people and teams, has been a celebration and just one example of how I've been able to develop my career.

Coaching is the universal language of change and learning, and as physiotherapists we don't always need to live in the realms of pathology and disease. Performance is unique and individual to everyone we meet, and coaching is crucial to achieving optimal performance. This is not just a sporting achievement; my coaching skills have heavily influenced my private practice and I strive each day to become a better coach to aid my patients in the best way I can.

Biggest Setbacks

Experience is a powerful teacher. Three simple strategies I used to aid this are being myself, building superstrengths and, most importantly, being open and honest. As I reflect on 8 fantastic years with British Paralympic swimming, one thing is clear: you can be a victim of change or a culprit. It's your choice! After the Rio Paralympic Games in 2016, my career hit a massive low. Two factors played a part. It was my first post-games blues, and the programme went through some challenging times from an athlete welfare perspective. We needed to work differently, to gain a better balance between athlete health and performance. As practitioners we must take the initiative where we see opportunity.

I read somewhere that you adapt, evolve, compete or die. I offered a solution and developed a nonclinical strategic role designed to redress the balance between performance and health. What we must remember is that out of adversity comes opportunity and a chance to be better. That is as relevant in the NHS as it is in private practice as it is in elite sport.

A Letter to My 80-Year-Old Self

First of all, I congratulate you on your achievements.

I just wish you had paid more attention earlier to your own self-belief over the beliefs and opinions of others. The energy wasted has been immense. Your plan worked out. You hit all your goals! But some goals are not meant to be hit. Did you honestly reach high enough? Did you take enough risks? Having said that, you didn't like being comfortable. I think part of the reason you've been successful is you've appreciated the importance of being uncomfortable. Proving people wrong and showing motivation and commitment to an outcome has probably been one of your greatest strengths but equally your greatest weakness; being so fixated on a plan at times has certainly led to living a socially sheltered life and at times feeling overwhelmed.

You needed to be better at maintaining contact with friends.

A Letter to My Disability

Thank you for giving me a purpose, to ensure I lived my life free from the expectations of others. My greatest achievement in life has been doing things people said I couldn't. Moving forward, I must remember the only thing that matters is my own opinion of myself and not to doubt the value I bring. My disability has often left me feeling alienated, and at times my life has been a challenge. But for every doubter there's been two supporters, and my support system has often dragged me through. Managing my disability will no doubt get tougher as I get older; when the time comes, I'll accept help and support when it's there and be grateful for it.

Reflections

Trust your gut.

Objectivity is also important. Sometimes people close to you know you better than you know yourself! But under no circumstances should they make the decision. It must be driven by you.

My Top Tips

Patient stories are more powerful than any objective test.

You can design the best rehabilitation plan there is, but if you have not involved the patient, how do you expect that to lead to long-term behaviour change? The big mistake a lot of people make is thinking education alone will lead to behaviour change. Unfortunately, this is not true. If working with athletes has taught me one thing, it's that often those who have experienced an injured state generally self-manage better in the future. On reflection, I think this is because I've been able to facilitate better understanding by helping them identify their past barriers to recovery and act on them using problem-solving skills specific to their experiences. I do this by building a solid therapeutic alliance. This is essential and is my top tip.

Stick to the plan, but don't be afraid to challenge it.

I know it's a bit of a cliché, but having an open and growth mindset is crucial. Physiotherapy is changing rapidly. What was in vogue yesterday will be gone tomorrow. We as physiotherapists must navigate these changing tides, and we do it more effectively with a mindset that allows honesty and evolution, honesty in the realisation that physiotherapy doesn't have all the answers and the ability to evolve with the changing evidence. It's OK to have more questions than answers. Having that open mindset will enable you to accept guidance and support to navigate through the ever-changing world of physiotherapy.

Finally, root cause analysis.

I want to share a process that has really shaped my practice, especially over the last 5 years. The '5 Whys' model was originally developed by Toyota. When we are faced with a problem, the solutions often present themselves after we've asked 'Why' five times. I find this useful in understanding barriers and challenges patients face when undertaking exercise programmes.

My 'Why'

I often get asked two questions: If I wasn't a physiotherapist, what would I be? And where do I see physiotherapy in the future? The first question is easy. I've never imagined a career other than working as a physiotherapist. I don't think you'll find a vocation that offers such a plethora of opportunities. More importantly, it is hugely rewarding. It really does feed my purpose. So where will we be in the future? There is so much out there around this, but I try to keep it simple. We will be what is required; how we get there depends on our ability to adapt, evolve and compete. Exercise and health promotion will be central to our services, as will our ability to see past pathology to the deeper psychosocial aspects of health. It's here where we can thrive.

Setbacks, Success, Personal Stories and Reflections – Deepak Agnihotri

Introduction

It's been a fascinating yet challenging journey from being an international physiotherapy student to being an advanced clinical practitioner to now working as the Director of Allied Health Professionals. I was born in India, where I did my undergraduate physiotherapy degree. My full training was for four and a half years. I wanted to work in the medical field, and one of the things that truly made me realise the potential of physiotherapy happened when I was placed in a hospital as a part of my internship. I went to an old age facility which was run by nuns, and the patient I was visiting only got out of bed once a day. I realised how rewarding it was when I saw the difference I could make in their life by being a physiotherapist. To this day, this remains the main motivation that I carry with me on my career journey as a physiotherapist.

The Journey

After qualifying, I worked in Mumbai, and then I came to the United Kingdom (UK) to do my postgraduate qualification. However, it was not so straightforward, as no one in my family had ever travelled abroad and they were worried and sceptical about my move to the UK. By that point my mentor and schoolteacher had taught me all about English – all aspects including language, literacy and grammar. He worked as a catalyst to convince my parents to allow me to go to the UK to pursue my dreams. My passion was gait analysis and manual therapy, and upon my research I found both were offered at the University of Salford. I was the only student in my cohort who got the vice chancellor's postgraduate scholarship, and it made me feel fortunate and proud when I received the gold student award. I completed MSc in advancing physiotherapy at the University of Salford Manchester and went on to work in clinical, research, education and leadership roles with four different National Health Service (NHS) trusts before moving to my role as training programme director (TPD) at NHS England (previously Health Education England). When I shared the news with my mentor about my TPD role, all he asked was that I 'help two individuals in life without asking for anything in return' and this would be his reward.

Getting My First Job in the NHS Was a Struggle

As an international physiotherapist, I had the clinical skills and knowledge, but I was not aware of the NHS system. I have been very fortunate with my university experience, as I got the opportunity to have a clinical placement in the NHS, supported by my personal tutor and head of school at the University of Salford Manchester.

Not knowing the NHS system or specific functions was the biggest challenge that I faced as an international student. I worked as a research associate and completed my dissertation on gait analysis. My first-ever research was published in 2014. After completing my MSc and research, my real career journey began. I filled in hundreds of applications and travelled to nearly every part of England for an interview by bus, train and motorbike. Finally the day came when I was offered a job in the NHS community. I clearly remember that day – I travelled to the interview on a motorbike, and halfway through the journey the rain came, and I arrived completely drenched. I went to a nearby charity shop and found a dry, clean shirt for the interview. That day I was finally successful, and my job search came to an end.

Lift as You Climb

I moved into the field of learning disability by chance when I was offered a band 6 job, fixed term, covering a maternity leave. Before this encounter, I didn't know that the role of physiotherapist specialising in learning disabilities existed. One of the things that struck me in the UK is that when you move into a field, you stay in that speciality, and you grow to make it your own and become a specialist in the space. The beauty of learning disabilities as a field is that I could use the full range of my skills and experiences in treating varied neurological, cardiorespiratory and musculoskeletal conditions. Working with people with learning disabilities is very rewarding, and soon making a difference in their lives became my passion, giving me happiness and satisfaction. However, I was supported massively by the members of the multidisciplinary team, including physiotherapy assistants. I learnt a lot from the physiotherapy assistants. In return, I was able to support my physiotherapy assistant to start on a physiotherapy apprentice programme. We both grew as part of this process, and I realised the actual meaning of 'lift as you climb'. I was growing but also lifting people along with me in my journey, which was beneficial to everyone.

Think Beyond Clinical

As I was growing, I realised that clinical skills are not enough to progress or to become successful as a physiotherapist. The support I got from my mentor and supervisors was very beneficial. I was encouraged to think beyond clinical and develop skills in leadership and research. As an advanced clinical practitioner, I work across the four pillars of advanced practice – clinical, research, education and leadership. On a typical day I see six or eight patients. The assessment and treatment sessions including nonmedical prescribing can take a lot longer due to communication issues and complex conditions. I could see service users at their home, in the hospital or in day centres. I often saw my patients over the span of a couple of months to help them achieve their goal and improve or maintain functional independence. I am passionate about quality improvement and clinical leadership provided by advanced clinical practitioners and providing innovative, evidence-based and person-centred care to people, meeting the needs of all our communities. I am the first independent prescriber-advanced clinical practitioner physiotherapist in the UK who is using prescribing skills and knowledge to help people with dementia and learning disabilities.

It's completely worth it when you see people acting independently, back on their feet with smiles on their faces; it feels so rewarding to see them enjoying life. It feels amazing when I hear about patients going on to lead active lives and families who feel supported by a person-centred plan. I worked as part of a multidisciplinary team which included nurses, doctors, a speech and language therapist, an occupational therapist, clinical psychologists, a physiotherapist and assistants. It was a great working environment, and we all supported one another to overcome any challenges in providing holistic care to our patients.

As a TPD, I did support trainee advanced practitioners and colleagues from diverse ethnicities and professional backgrounds to become successful advanced practitioners while working across the four pillars. I then took the leadership role as national clinical advisor for learning disabilities and autism. I worked strategically at the local, regional and national levels in collaboration with other stakeholders and professional bodies to make a positive impact, demonstrating the value of the role of advanced practitioner and nonmedical consultants in delivering person-centred care for people with learning disability and autistic people.

Networking Is Key

I once attended a conference in London, and I was not very confident. I did not know anyone before I entered the venue. However, through networking at the conference I spoke to senior NHS leaders and built professional relationships. Networking helped me explore opportunities that I may not have considered. As a result of networking, I came to know about the opportunity to lead a national project at Health Education England. After being successful in getting the job, I led on the ethical and sustainable international recruitment of allied health professionals at Health Education England. I worked strategically at the national level in collaboration with other stakeholders and professional bodies to make a positive impact, demonstrating the value of the role of allied health professional and advanced clinical practitioner.

Networking helps in gaining the confidence to communicate effectively and succinctly as a leader. I have worked as a member of the Black Asian Minority Ethnic (BAME) Allied Health Professions Strategic Advisor at NHS England. I then became the chair of BAME+ network, which is now called Diversity Alliance Network, in my last NHS trust. I am honoured to have won an award in October 2020 for outstanding contribution to the work of equality, diversity and inclusion from the Royal College of Nursing Northwest in celebration of Black History Month. Through networking, I also got a job as a visiting lecturer teaching trainee advanced practitioner at the Higher Education Institute in northwest England.

As Director of Allied Health Professionals, I utilise all my my experience and networking skills to continue a culture of openness and honesty to demonstrate that diverse leadership is critical to a thriving NHS.

A Final Few Words

The NHS is the best organisation I have ever seen and worked for. I've been particularly impressed with the services that are offered. It is amazing to see that we recognise the major role that physiotherapy can play in improving people's quality of life. I would recommend a career in physiotherapy to anyone, as it offers endless opportunities, great job satisfaction and work-life balance. It's a very good profession that teaches you specialist skills that you can use to make a difference in someone's life.

My Top Three Tips

1. Always think about four pillars of practice: clinical, research, education and leadership.
2. Lift as you climb.
3. Networking is the key to growth.

Setbacks, Success, Personal Stories and Reflections – Evert Verhagen

Introduction

When I was younger, my father took me to local running events, and I have been a runner ever since. I competed at the national level as a junior, finishing fifth in cross-country and tenth in middle-distance events. A knee injury prevented me from continuing at that level, so I decided to study human movement sciences to better understand what happened to me. So, before you continue reading, let's get this out of the way: I am not a physiotherapist. I am a lecturer and researcher with over 25 years of experience in epidemiology, prevention and rehabilitation of musculoskeletal complaints in active and inactive populations. My research focuses on preventing sports and physical activity-related injuries, including monitoring, cost-effectiveness and implementation issues. I have supervised multiple (inter-) national PhDs and postdocs, including physiotherapists, and have (co-)authored nearly 400 peer-reviewed publications.

Reflecting Back and Forth

These are always difficult questions to answer because they get to the heart of the matter: Would you do things differently if you could go back in time? I would not have made a single different decision in my life or career. Setbacks and circumstances are part of who I am as a person. If you allow yourself to acknowledge them, you will learn. My current life lessons to my younger self would centre on this idea: Live. Go out there. Show yourself. Make mistakes. It is all fine. You lose some, but you also gain some. It's all a part of life, and it is wonderful. I wonder, though, whether my 8-year-old self would understand such a philosophical message.

If I was looking back on my career from a much older age, I would be asking questions humbly. What is the best career path for me to take? What decisions have I come to regret? Will I be able to live a happy life? We probably all want to know the answers to these questions in a quest to live a better, more fulfilling life. However, this is a clear case of the grass being greener on the other side. After all, once we know which pitfalls to avoid and which paths to take, once we are at a certain age, we likely come to regret certain decisions anyway.

159

Career Ups and Downs

SETBACKS

I see opportunities rather than setbacks. Naturally, I had amazing ideas for scientific projects and wrote, in my opinion, the best manuscript of the decade, but I received rejections, and it still hurts. I have started mentoring students for whom, in retrospect, I may not have been the best mentor. I feel like I let those students down. I could go on and on about such 'mistakes' that may have hampered or delayed my career progress, but I would not call them setbacks. Such intentions may have hampered my career advancement at that specific time, but the lessons learnt from such engagements paid off later.

However, using the term 'setback' broadly, I will bring up a point about mentorship and supervision. When I first began my academic career, I was mentored by a highly acclaimed professor. I am grateful to him for his lessons and advice. On the other hand, his presence has slowed my advancement as an individual professional. As a junior, you are generally guided by a more experienced and well-connected senior peer. Instead of being mentored, my work and ideas were presented as my mentor's rather than mine. It took me a long time to carve out a place for myself in our realm, aside from anger and frustration and possibly a broken friendship. The takeaway is that you must have the courage to speak up when being mentored. Step out from under their shadow. As a mentor, you must also provide a safe environment in which to engage in constructive dialogue.

SUCCESSES

How do you define success? A 'success' for me is simply something I am proud of. I am proud, for instance, when a PhD student successfully defends their thesis. I am especially proud when this student has a practical background, such as a physical therapist, because I believe in the connection between science and practice. We need practice to ask meaningful questions and science to answer those questions. Consider the possibility of wearing both hats.

I am pleased when someone takes an idea I had in the past and expands on it. For example, I was once asked to write a text about the physical therapist's role in promoting physical activity for health. I had forgotten about this text until years later when I was contacted by a student therapist who had read my ideas and wanted to create a study based on them. This felt like a success.

If I had to pick one accomplishment, it would be my appointment as a university research chair, a prestigious position that is granted once a year. I was nominated, which I already consider a personal success. That is, someone believes I am qualified for such a position. I had to defend my research ideas and projected societal impact before a committee. I decided to present myself and my goals. There was to be no sugar-coating; take me or leave me! That year, I was the only one to receive this honourable position: a professional victory and a personal win.

A Personal Story

One turning point in my career taught me a lot. I stayed in academia after finishing my PhD. I stayed in academia after finishing my PhD. Through my research, I hoped to make a positive difference in clinical practice and assist both clinicians and patients. I quickly discovered that the academic game is not played in this manner. Grants are required to conduct research. Instead of finding grants that suit your question, you must find questions that fit a grant opportunity. Those are not always the questions that are relevant for practice, so I decided to leave academia and try to make a difference somewhere else. I got a job at a municipal health department. I oversaw the epidemiological department and was responsible for guiding policy based on the local public health situation. I was completely at ease when I first started. I got to conduct research, write practical implications and supervise the implementation of the given advice. In theory, yes. In practice, everything was completely different. I had to leverage different priorities and political agendas and priorities. In the end, very little of my advice was taken seriously. It was a complete waste of my time and energy. I yearned for the freedom and a sense of purpose that academic research provided. It took this adventure outside the university walls to realise this and understand my worth as an academic researcher in practice. Fortunately, I still had a foot in the door at university and could find my way back. I vowed to conduct research that I believed would benefit sports practice.

My Advice to Newcomers in the Profession

'Knowledge is the eye of desire and can become the pilot of the soul', Will Durant said. This quote applies to any profession, but I have seen it apply to physical therapists. It is easy to read a textbook or a (pseudo) scientific text, accept that knowledge as gospel and live by it, for example, following the 'hype' treatments that have appeared. In general, such treatments are not well supported by research. Their acceptance is typically driven by a small group of authoritative therapists who vouch for it or by industry, which uses a well-funded marketing campaign to sell a product. Furthermore, finding a quote on social media and accepting it as truth is simple.

Never take knowledge for granted. Maintain your curiosity and never be afraid to ask questions. Physical therapy is a profession that is constantly evolving and changing. Research yields new insights daily. Be open to new developments and continue to expand your knowledge and expertise as you advance professionally. This means that you must sometimes accept evidence or knowledge that contradicts your own beliefs or experiences. To be honest, my academic background influences my opinion. A physical therapist is endowed with a basic understanding of science. This enables you to evaluate new knowledge not only on its face value but also on its internal and external validity.

There is no need to master scientific skills, but it is necessary to understand the limitations and importance of the evidence presented. I usually compare it to macarons, a sweet meringue-based confection. The recipe is deceptively simple, with few ingredients. However, the steps involved in combining these ingredients to create delectable sweets necessitate experience and skill. Make no attempt to bake macarons. Let the professionals handle it. However, understand what makes a good macaron and enjoy them accordingly. The same is true for science.

Things I Wish I Had Known Before I Started

At the start of my career as an academic researcher, I wish someone had told me how important it was to have a strong support system. I learnt along the way the benefit of having family, friends and co-workers who provide feedback and encouragement in my work.

Also, it would have been helpful to have proper mentor who provided guidance and advice on navigating the academic environment successfully. This mentor could have taught me the value of investing in networking and developing relationships with other professionals, both in my academic field and in other fields. This would have allowed me to gain important insights into the process of conducting meaningful research for practice. I would have been able to construct a powerful professional network, which is critical for progressing in one's career.

I wish I had been more aware of the significance of caring for oneself. It is easy to feel overburdened by the requirements of your professional life; therefore, it is essential to take breaks and put one's own health and happiness as a top priority. It is essential to practice self-care not only to preserve your physical and mental health but also to retain your focus and maximise the quality of your work.

I wish I had known to keep myself organised. To ensure that tasks are finished promptly, it is essential to have a method in place for staying organised regarding deadlines.

Final Reflections

Looking back on my personal and professional development, I am filled with pride and accomplishment.

I have been fortunate enough to have mentors and colleagues who have pushed me to be the best I can be. I have been able to take on more responsibility, learn new skills and take on leadership roles. I have also taken the time to expand my knowledge through training, courses and reading materials. Through this, I have become a well-informed professional, able to make informed decisions and tackle difficult tasks. In my personal life, I have dedicated time to building relationships with people and forming meaningful connections. I have learnt to appreciate the small moments and cherish the time spent with friends and family. I have also tried to focus on gratitude, recognising the importance of being thankful for the good in my life. I have also worked hard to care for my physical and mental health, understanding the importance of self-care.

Setbacks, Success, Personal Stories and Reflections – Roisin McNulty

Introduction

I am a sports and musculoskeletal physiotherapist working around sport and performance environments for the past 15 years. I've always loved sports. My siblings and I played everything we could as kids – soccer, rounders, basketball, tennis, Gaelic football, obstacle races and gymnastics – whatever we could make up and always competitive. On winter Saturday mornings we were glued to ski jumping on Eurosport (we had never been near a ski slope in our lives but were assured experts).

Having sampled many sports, I took up judo at age 10 and it clicked. That was it for me. I was half-decent at it and it became a huge part of my life for the next 10 years. I made the Irish team, and despite a leg infection that put me in hospital for 10 days in the summer of 1999, I competed at the Youth Olympics 3 weeks later. It was an exhilarating experience but ultimately devastating not to perform to what I believed were my capabilities. I left with an appetite for being around high-performance environments that would stay with me.

Whilst growing up, I lived next door to a sports physician, Dr. Paul Sandys. My sister and I would call in to Paul frequently after a mishap at judo training, desperate to compete the coming weekend. My father used to mow his lawn and give him some meat from the farm in return. I am certain we got the better deal. Paul taught me about anatomy and rehab and gave me sports medicine books so that I could read up on my injuries. I devoured every bit and therein began my learning journey of the body. Paul also gave me books on mindset and psychology, and I know these shaped me hugely as an impressionable young teenager. He was an amazing man, very generous with his energy and quite ahead of his time.

Why This?

Human skills are fundamental to physiotherapy practice, and I was delighted to hear this resource was being put together. I have always been intrigued by the connection and interaction piece of physiotherapy, of listening to people's stories and unravelling the puzzle. I think as physios, we are in such a privileged position and the power of our words cannot be underestimated. The subjective examination has always been a particular piece of interest to me, honed from the fishbowl sessions during my clinical master's.

Nothing like this book existed when I was studying or early in my career. I also had no idea about the 'outside the box' opportunities that exist in physiotherapy, and I hope sharing them can help open some eager physiotherapist's eyes to the possibilities.

Range

I took the scenic route to physiotherapy, and in hindsight, it served a lot of 'range', a term coined by David Epstein. My academic journey started at the University of Galway in 2000 in the bachelor of commerce programme, which didn't stick. The content did not inspire me, and I dropped out after 1 year. With nothing in place for the next year, I managed to claim a last-minute spot on a 12-month sports and recreation leadership certificate programme and there began my formal studies in sport. We had some fantastic teachers on the course who fuelled my passion for sport and performance. I got my coaching certificates and learned the fundamentals of training and injury management. It set me up well to commence a degree in sport and exercise science at the University of Limerick (UL) the following year. The years at UL were formative and I found myself particularly interested in biomechanics and S&C (strength & conditioning). I took the opportunity to go to Australia during the third-year placement. Grand plans of doing my placement at a new academy of sport fell apart 2 weeks before I was due to go. I said nothing, jumped on the plane and figured I would make something work when I got there. As luck would have it, a teammate at Sydney University Rugby Club managed a gym in Sydney. She gave me a job, which served the criteria for the university placement, and I used my spare time to shadow at sports physiotherapy clinics and at Manly Rugby Club on match days. It was after this experience that I realised physiotherapy was what I wanted to pursue.

Upon graduating from UL I spent 12 months with UL Bohemians (Bohs) Rugby Academy (a team based in Limerick, in Midwest Ireland) in a support S&C role, juggling with girls rugby development work for the Connacht Rugby Branch (the Rugged, west of Ireland). The physiotherapy itch was ready to be scratched, and after a 12-month break from studying, I enrolled in the graduate physiotherapy programme at University of Sydney. Fast-forward a few years and I had come full circle, now working in a clinic at the University of New South Wales, where I had shadowed 5 years earlier. Dr Mark Stewart was a fantastic mentor, and we had a great team of young, motivated physiotherapists in the clinic. It was an amazing learning environment and we saw everything from high-level student athletes to weekend warriors to miserable PhD students with neck and back pain from too many hours in front of the laptop. Keen to refine my practice, I enrolled in the master of musculoskeletal and sports physiotherapy programme at Griffith University in 2013, a challenging and very worthwhile undertaking.

The Rugby Chapter

When I started at UL, I moved in with a group of girls who played rugby. The college team were short of players for an upcoming 7s tournament in France, and when they heard I did judo they weren't long roping me in. Two training sessions later, I'm on the college team trip, loving every minute and enjoying the comradery that a team sport offered. The three trips per week back to Galway for judo training were soon swapped out for rugby. I improved as a player, solidified a position in the UL Bohs team and got a few provincial seasons under my belt with Connacht and Munster. When I moved to Australia, I joined the Sydney University side, and as my physiotherapy studies commenced I was provided with the perfect opportunity for learning within the club. With little to no support for women's rugby at that time, I was playing the roles of team physiotherapist and player. It was a fantastic learning experience, and I was exposed to a lot of acute traumatic injuries on the spot. Over time, as my experience grew and I developed good working relationships with coaches, players and doctors, I found physiotherapy opportunities with representative teams. This led to the appointment as team physiotherapist for the Australia women's rugby team, the Wallaroos, for the 2014 Women's Rugby World Cup campaign. The programme was not professional at the time, and we came together for camps and a couple of tours before the World Cup. I'm thrilled to see the progress the programme has made in the past years and the support that has since developed for the women's game.

The Circus Chapter

As fate would go, I won tickets to a Cirque du Soleil show when I was studying physiotherapy in Sydney. I had never heard of Cirque and could barely believe my eyes. I thought it was the most incredible thing I had ever seen. Sometime after, I heard about a physiotherapist that was joining Cirque to work full-time. It had never entered my head that physiotherapists might work in such an environment. Roll on 7 years, with my clinical masters completed, I was keen for a change from the combination of clinic and rugby. I wanted to work full-time in sport or performance and, with a thirst for travel, I remembered Cirque. I saw they had positions open and got in touch. What followed came unbelievably fast. Within 3 weeks of writing a letter, I had an offer and had 1 month to move to Montreal for the launch of a new production. I knew I could not let the opportunity pass me by and Nelly packed her bags. I arrived in Montreal in the early hours of a January morning, −20°, a far cry from the Sydney summer I had just left. I had 24 hours to find a winter coat and boots and report to international HQ. What unfolded over the next four-and-a-half years was an incredible personal and professional journey. There was a lot to learn, from understanding demands of the different performer roles to navigating working for a large corporation. It was overwhelming at times, and on occasion I asked myself what the hell I was doing there. Thankfully, I was reassured it was normal to feel out of your depth in the first year and it was a great lesson in getting comfortable with discomfort. The show went on the road after an intensive 4-month preparation, and then we moved from city to city every week. Over the next 4 years we made our way through North America, Europe, Russia and Central and South America. My passport collected many stamps!

It's hard to describe the mix of experiences you encounter when travelling with a 'family' of 100 people, week in and week out, coming together to put something spectacular on a stage and dealing with the random things that pop up like a hurricane and evacuation in Florida in 2018 or a major power cut across three countries in South America in 2019 (we still performed two shows that day). It was a real-life lesson in collaboration, and I loved it. Solving problems around injuries often involved getting out of the 'physiotherapist box' and consulting other departments such as wardrobe or stage management. It was fun to bring the scientific piece to that environment and at the same time to be prepared to find middle ground with the other stakeholders. Where possible we always tried to keep the performer in the show in some capacity, even if doing very light cues.

The COVID-19 pandemic put a stop to our lives in March 2020, and little did we know how long that stop would be. With many friends back on the road now, I find myself somewhat of a Cirque groupie in 2023, catching the shows in Europe and getting my old tour-life fix one weekend at a time.

Setbacks

As the neurolinguistic programming (NLP) presupposition goes, 'There is no failure, only feedback', or as John Maxwell puts it, 'Sometimes you win, sometimes you learn'. This theme has been very true for me over the years, and whilst there was no shortage of setbacks, in hindsight there always seemed to be a lesson in it or something else on my path that was better than what I could imagine.

There were numerous jobs I went for where I was unsuccessful, from my planned internship at an academy of sport during my sport science studies to a new-grad position at the National Coaching and Training Center at UL and various applications to professional jobs in rugby and other sports where I didn't get so much as an acknowledgement email. I didn't get into my first-choice physiotherapy school; I only got into my clinical master's because someone declined their offer and it was only my willingness to learn that got me in. Upon receiving a letter of rejection, I wrote to the convener of the programme and asked him for feedback on how I could improve my application for the next intake. Three days later I got a call from the admissions office saying someone had declined and my name was on the list of people to call.

The lessons learned from athlete care always sting. There came a moment when I confronted the harsh reality of misjudging a performer's inconclusive concussion assessment. Driven by my own internal pressure, and a rush to make a decision, I cleared him to continue, on the rationale that he wasn't involved in any risky feats, only for him to return to my door with an exacerbation of symptoms 2 hours later. I will never know, but what might have been a straightforward recovery stretched into a gruelling 5 weeks. The individual played a pivotal role, and the situation placed an additional burden on numerous team members. To be explicitly clear, the company has stringent protocols for concussion management; this error was solely mine. There was nothing to do but accept responsibility and learn from it. The experience stayed with me thereafter, prompting me to incorporate this scenario as a crucial interview question in subsequent interviews I conducted.

A Rollercoaster Has Ups and Downs

Getting into physiotherapy school felt like a huge success for me. I was thrilled. I remember feeling proud and excited to be a physiotherapist, as I had always admired physiotherapists through my own sporting endeavours.

Some obvious career highs were being appointed as the Wallaroos physiotherapist, which felt like a huge achievement, and getting the job at Cirque, which felt like a dream.

Whilst the positions themselves were recognition of the work I had put in, the day-to-day experience of those environments, collaborating with incredible people and the wins along the way in supporting performers are the things that keep you going. Performers telling you months later how much of a difference you made to them, that is where the real sense of reward came.

Selected Personal Stories

Cirque provided some interesting scenarios where I would find myself wondering, 'How on earth did I get here?':

1. If you can't beat them …
   We had a group of Russian and Ukrainian 'strongmen'. Their role was to throw the female fliers to each other and catch them (on podiums elevated over 4 m above the stage). Their main act was at the end of the first half of the show, and during intermission it wasn't unusual to find them competing in the gym. This somehow progressed to arm wrestling competitions. I walked into the physiotherapy room one day to find 10 men, in full makeup and tight insect costumes, yelling and cheering each other on in an arm wrestling competition. Turns out the up-down bed was particularly favourable for getting the correct height. I told them they needed to take it elsewhere – if they were going to arm wrestle, I didn't want to be witness to one of them rupturing something in my treatment room. Fast-forward 3 days later and I return to a similar scenario with my physiotherapy colleague in the middle of the competition. I gave up trying to stop it and joined the cheer squad for that one.

2. 'Don't get too ahead of yourself'.

We ran a project with lots of departments on our show to reduce the injury burden of one group of acrobats. We appeared to have some success with a few initiatives, and I proudly presented our project findings at the Performance Medicine Summit later that year. I finished my presentation to a good round of applause, thinking we really nailed it. But 15 minutes later I received a message saying that two of the performers in that group had sustained an Achilles tear and plantar fascia rupture that very day, bringing me back to earth rather quickly and instantly killing any sense of 'I have this all figured out'!

3. 'Things aren't always as they appear'.

The 'image does not reflect function' conversation was never more obvious than at Cirque. I will never forget seeing the spinal X-rays of a performer who was doing remarkably complex acrobatics without significant symptoms, nor the doctor's face when he saw the X-rays! Another acrobat could perform a triple back somersault on an airtrack with the scrawniest Achilles tendon you've ever seen. A botched surgery from years earlier and no specific rehabilitation meant that whilst he couldn't do one single calf raise, he could still somehow compensate and do some incredibly explosive jumping. The power of the body to adapt is truly remarkable (but yes, we put him on a calf-strengthening programme).

Being a Chameleon, Ever-Changing Colours and Adapting to New Environments

I have always been somewhat of a chameleon and enjoy new challenges. Working in the fast-paced and creative environments of Cirque du Soleil and more recently Red Bull Athlete Performance fostered a passion to seek innovative solutions in my work and to ask the question 'What if'. The COVID-19 pandemic allowed time for reflection and offered some space to explore concepts around design thinking and needs-led innovation. Inspired by some of the amazing work going on in broader healthcare fields, my next adventure will take me a little further outside the traditional physiotherapy realm.

The transferable skills innate to physiotherapists, such as problem solving, having a patient-centred focus and working in a team, are taking me to the BioInnovate Fellowship at the University of Galway. The programme is based on the Stanford BioDesign model, which is a proven method for innovation in the medical field. I hope to represent the profession well as I collaborate with doctors, engineers and business experts to identify unmet needs in clinical areas and create meaningful solutions.

Key Reflections on My Career Journey

My biggest reflections are that (1) there are learning opportunities everywhere, sometimes where you least expect it, and (2) the outcome is not the outcome; the end is not the end (taken from the parable of the farmer and the horse – worth a read).

1. Learning is everywhere.

There was a lot of value in certain roles that I didn't appreciate at the time. I grafted and did a lot of sports coverage without payment whilst a student, learning from experienced practitioners. Doing gigs with recreational athletes, like overseeing the physiotherapy coverage of the UNSW team of 500 athletes at Australian Uni Games, really taught me how to plan a mobile clinic and organise a medical referral network on the move – these skills were crucial for my time at Cirque.

2. The outcome is not the outcome.

Things change, goalposts move and what was the perfect job or experience at age 25 will be different at age 35. Sometimes learnings or setbacks are setting you up for something bigger, better and more rewarding. What was most important and served me well was to keep learning, adapting and moving forward.

What I Would Tell 8-Year-Old Roisin

You can't even imagine the things you will do and people you will meet; anything really is possible. Just enjoy the ride and soak up every moment (cliché, I know, but true). Enjoy time with great teachers and write things down!

My Three Pieces of Advice to Newcomers in the Profession

1. Go get experience and don't expect to be paid for all of it.
   This is a hot topic, and it may be an unpopular opinion. I recognise that this can be abused, and it is a hot debate in the S&C profession. I'm not suggesting full-time 40 hours-a-week internships that are unpaid, but getting experience and learning from practitioners by offering an extra set of hands was invaluable to me. There are many things you only learn on the job and getting the chance to learn and refine these skills in a supported environment is important.
2. Learn from other professions.
   S&C coaches, sport scientists and psychologists have incredible skills that are all relevant to a good sports physiotherapist. The more you can understand the different perspectives, the more well rounded your approach can be.
3. Stay curious and open minded.
   You will come to realise that the more you learn, the less you know. I felt significantly less assured about my knowledge after my clinical master's than I did after my physiotherapy degree!

What I Would Whisper to 80-Year-Old Roisin

The outcome was not the outcome, the end was not the end … and life was only beginning at 40!

Setbacks, Success, Personal Stories and Reflections – Evangelos Benatos and Andreas Gatzoulis

Introduction (Written Predominantly by Evangelos)

Undoubtedly in our profession, apart from the essential clinical, knowledge and expertise skills, we must possess strong so-called soft skills which will ultimately play a dramatic role in our personal and professional career journeys. Healthcare is an amazing field of practice, unique and competitive, precisely because of the individuality of every human being, whether they are healthcare providers or patients. The right balance between the hard and soft skills is what drives healthcare professionals to have long-lasting and successful careers.

My personal journey started as a young kid who really enjoyed playing outdoors. In the early 2000s my friends and I would still gather at our neighbourhood park to play all kinds of games and sports until it was too late or too dark to be outside. My favourite sport was always soccer, so from age 8 till age 22 I played at an amateur level. The only times I didn't enjoy myself as much were the times when I needed to be on the sidelines due to injury or illness. However, it was during these times that I discovered my spark to become involved with healthcare and more specifically to become a physiotherapist. Even though I didn't know it at the time, I was amazed by the process and the procedure of getting an athlete (professional or amateur) back to their previous healthy state and athletic duties. So at age 18 I enrolled in the University of Thessaly, Greece, in the Department of Physiotherapy.

My First Role With a Professional Club

While I was a student and amateur soccer player, I received a job offer to join the city's local team which was then competing at the second national division. It is common in Greece for nonelite or subelite sports teams to recruit soon-to-graduate students or recently graduated physiotherapists, as they may offer low salaries but also provide work experience and the opportunity to build a reputation and enhance CVs. Without a second thought, mostly for the reasons written above, I accepted the opportunity to start working with the professional team. I accepted with enthusiasm, hoping that this could someday provide the ticket to something bigger and better. I have always been like this, weighing the pros and cons of the choices I make and trying to make the most of each opportunity with my eyes on what may come next.

Adapting to the new environment wasn't difficult for me. Although levels were unmatched and incomparable, I felt my previous experience as a player gave me an advantage in understanding a player's mindset. Also, the fact that the team wasn't a major competitor gave me much-needed time to learn. At the time my role was to provide first aid for on-field injuries, soft tissue work, ankle taping and mobility stretching. For the most part the players would refer to a private physiotherapy clinic for anything more than muscle soreness. I voluntarily worked at a clinic as well, as I wanted to be present from the moment of injury to the moment the player returned to play.

I have always been a quick learner and knowledge enthusiast. Being able to solve puzzles and problems excites me, so being in this environment working with professional athletes in the morning and everyday people in the afternoon gave me the desire to continue to become a better overall clinician. The opportunity meant I was able to practice and enhance my communication and social skills with people from different backgrounds who were each aiming for individual outcomes and goals.

The Importance of Soft Skills

A real turning point for me was when I recognised the importance of being a good listener. It is important to listen carefully to the patient not only to derive crucial information about an injury but also to understand the patient's psychosocial state, which is of equivalent, if not greater, importance. This made me more compassionate and helped me see things from a different point of view, where there is not only a given injury but also a person behind this injury, and we as clinicians should treat the person first and foremost.

My growing knowledge and experience as well as my personality earned me the trust of the head physiotherapist and the team's front office too, which in turn gave me greater responsibilities as time went by. Eventually, however, I had to resign from my position to serve my military duty, which is obligatory for every Greek man over age 18. After that, I faced the biggest challenge of my professional career: I got a job at Olympiacos Basketball Club, a prestigious and historic club that competes in the highest-level tier professional club basketball competition in Europe, the EuroLeague. By the way, this happens to be the club I have supported since I was a young child.

Rising to Meet Higher Expectations

The level of professionalism I encountered there was something I had never seen before. I quickly realised I would need to rise to live up to the new expectations. My biggest challenge was to settle and integrate myself into a team that was experiencing and is still experiencing great success and has some of the best elite basketball players while being the newcomer and the youngest member of the staff – younger than some of the players. At first, what helped me through this situation was my patience. I had faith in myself and my abilities and knowledge, but my intention was not to show off just because I felt I could. My goal was for players and my co-workers to become accustomed to my presence and then to gain their trust through small steps. I was always available for whoever needed, always happy to share my opinion whenever it was asked and more than competent to help the team achieve their goals through my work. Opportunities soon arrived not only to showcase my working skills arsenal but also to showcase that I am trustworthy and loyal, which is highly anticipated and appreciated.

At this level of competition, even the smallest details can play a major part in a team's success, and winning or losing often comes down to the last second of a game. So both inside and outside the court, I tried to maintain mental and psychological stability which in the end helped me manage stress levels and enabled me to make better decisions – both of which are crucial professionally and personally. As backroom staff, what we needed was to maintain a great level of communication between us and the players.

Communication as Key to Success

Working in an environment which involves many people is quite challenging. Each person is different and has a personal life and personal troubles. Opinions and beliefs may vary, which can often produce friction and arguments. Communication between the players, head coach, assistant coaches, backroom staff, S&C (strength & conditioning) coaches and medical staff, as a group or individually, was crucial to success. What I tried to do was to always be myself, true and loyal to everyone but, at the same time, accept that we are a team and everything should happen for the greater good. It took me two seasons to fully adapt to my new reality, the new expectations and the new needs.

Final Thoughts

Currently, I am in my fourth season in Olympiacos, internally promoted as the head physiotherapist of the team, and have gotten a place in the medical staff of the National Men's Basketball team of Greece since last summer. To this day, I have never stopped trying to be a better version of myself personally and professionally. I have been studying hard, following recent literature and trying to implement new things while also working on the vital soft skills. I have finally settled myself as a strong healthcare provider, and I have built strong personal relationships with my colleagues based on mutual respect, loyalty and honesty.

Setbacks, Success, Personal Stories and Reflections – Chris Jones

Introduction

When I was first invited to write a chapter regarding my experience of becoming a sport and exercise medicine (SEM) consultant, my immediate response was, 'Oh I don't think so'. I felt my chest tighten. It was how I remember feeling when as a 15-year-old I was asked to be head boy of our school. An intense fear of being – in any way – the centre of attention. David (an editor of the book), inspiring as ever, was relaxed. 'No pressure', he said. 'Write a few words about your journey and we can take it from there'. So here we go.

Setbacks

In SEM we can take on multiple roles, with sports teams or at several clinics, developing a 'portfolio of work'. We are the ideal practitioners to work within and lead multidisciplinary teams for musculoskeletal medicine and physical activity initiatives. However, our roles within the public health sector require further expansion and investment. The challenges we face include demonstrating our worth to other specialists who have in previous years led these services.

Community-based programmes can help improve physical activity. Walk with a Doc is an American-inspired organisation where physicians lead a walk for patients and participants after a quick group educational health talk. A mentor's son suggested we set this up at our clinic. It was inspiring and I was excited to set up our own Walk with a Doc in Regents Park, London. Sadly, such an initiative requires much more marketing and investment of energy than we were able to deliver. Some patients came but numbers were smaller than envisioned, and I had the feeling they were only coming to support me rather than themselves. As the cold, wet days of winter approached, the number of participants dropped. It was a flop! On reflection, I was surprised local communities did not use the service despite extensive networking with local general practitioners (GPs). This challenge was a low point but one that I hope will have a resurgence in future.

The Availability Challenge

There are constant challenges in our work, which keeps us motivated to learn and succeed. The amount of availability required in sports medicine roles can be challenging.

I recall having a disagreement with a football club manager where I was club doctor. My role was part-time: one session a week and home match day cover. I explained that there was no way I could cover a last-minute friendly match, but I could tell he was excited as it was against Premier League opposition. To cover the match, I would have needed to cancel all my clinic commitments, so I explained I was not prepared to make such last-minute changes. Over previous seasons, I had spoken to the club to recommend additional doctor support. I had slowly begun to take on more responsibility than initially contracted. Financial restraints and club ownership changes were the apparent reason for a lack of doctor cover. The academy did not have regular doctor support and I felt obliged to help support these young prospects. Football managers are rarely refused anything within the club; unfortunately, however, everyone has a varying tolerance of what they will and will not accept.

Successes

One major achievement was having my application for certificate of eligibility for specialist registration (CESR) in sport and exercise medicine accepted. It certainly was not the smoothest of routes into the speciality. It is an alternative route to the traditional SEM training programme into gaining recognition as an SEM consultant. It involves collecting an expansive portfolio of work over several years and matching this to the curriculum of the training programme. My advice to younger doctors is to apply for the training programme which is well structured and organised.

There is very good exposure to the curriculum topics, and ultimately everyone involved wants you to succeed. Taking the CESR route feels like the opposite. At times it felt impossible to meet the curriculum requirements. Communication with the GMC is a long, tiring journey, and without the support of others it is not an easy feat. I am truly grateful to everyone who has helped in this process. If anyone reading this is considering a CESR application, I wish you well and I am very happy to offer my support with your journey.

Finding Balance for Success

The key to success is finding the role (or roles) where you are happiest. Success in our family, social or work life requires balance. SEM can be competitive, and certainly some of the roles can affect family life. Roles in sports teams, for example, often impact weekends, involve trips abroad and carry unsociable hours. Team doctors must interrupt things at the drop of a hat to provide the necessary care to players.

I love sports and have loved being a team doctor for a couple of professional football clubs over seven seasons. Watching sports and ultimately being paid at the same time certainly fed my inner joy. I loved the buzz around weekend matches. But despite my roles only being part-time, they still at times had the power to become domineering. How much the role impacts the rest of your life is dependent on the club's medical setup, the agreements in place and ultimately what you are prepared to be involved in – potentially for no extra earnings. Being involved in Charlton Athletic's promotion from League One to the English Championship at Wembley Stadium in London was an unforgettable experience. The lows of an own goal after 5 minutes but then the highs of a stoppage time winner. It was electric.

Trophies and promotion are successes for the whole team and club. However, day-to-day successes, such as when players return to play after a difficult injury or illness, give me a deeper sense of fulfilment and pride.

Unmatched Experiences

Working in an SEM clinic full-time provides access to incredible rehabilitation facilities and highly trained staff. Over the years this has exposed me to some amazing cases.

I have witnessed patients who are pre-diabetic coming into the clinic and transforming their metabolic profile. I have worked with patients with other health comorbidities such as cancer, cardiovascular disease and psychological ill health who wish to find comfort and health changes through exercise. It is a proven method of medicine. Successes such as these are no less significant than winning matches and trophies with sports clubs.

We support the transformation of a patient's lifestyle in the hope that they will live a longer, happier and healthier life with their loved ones. They trust us as sport and exercise advocates to help them achieve their goals. There is nothing remarkable about the concept. It is simply an exercise programme that we prescribe and support.

I am at a stage where I am starting to see ex-patients with different injuries and their friends and family members. Is there any bigger reward than having someone recommend their loved one to you?.

It was not until David suggested I write this chapter that I reflected on what I love most about my role. It is the egalitarianism and importance of exercise as medicine. The leading risk of non-communicable disease is physical inactivity. More than a quarter of the world's adult population are insufficiently active (https://www.who.int/news-room/fact-sheets/detail/physical-activity). It's our duty as sport and exercise doctors to support society and reduce the impact on healthcare systems. We can be involved from policy level to community level. Every aspect of this is potentially rewarding.

At this moment in my life, I've moved away from professional club sport. I enjoy having the weekends with my family and time away from work. Despite the fact that I am a GP and an SEM consultant, it was not until we had our twins that I began to feel any emotional attachment to key development stages. Watching them learn to crawl, walk, swim, ride bikes and begin to develop technical skills in sport is incredible. These 'smaller' successes are immeasurable.

Personal Stories

Working with professionals and celebrities can lead to inevitable friendships, developing through reduced formality in varying work settings. But no matter who you are caring for, it is vital to remember that you are the patient's health professional and as such have a responsibility to always maintain professional standards.

Recently, an ex-professional footballer raised a legal case against an orthopaedic surgeon, an alleged negligence claim. The player unfortunately did not recover to the level of performance he wanted following knee surgery. Without going into specifics, the player blamed the surgeon for a complication. The claim was brought forward several years after the player's surgery, as he continued to play at a lower level. I had been the player's club doctor at the time of surgery. I had been the player's advocate, in a sense, his friend. I also knew the surgeon, who is excellent. The whole situation was stressful for everyone involved. All our communications were shared with legal teams: emails, phone calls, text message conversations and medical records. A tremendous amount of money was involved in the case, and so it went to the high court. I was called in as a witness. Everything was scrutinised. Trying to make sense of conversations recorded in notes from several years before was a sobering experience.

The experience shone a harsh spotlight on how crucial it is to take precise notes. To our credit as a medical department, we were successful in this. Time is precious and shifts at work can be busy, yet every single word we record in the medical notes has the possibility of being cross-examined. For example, 'Why did you use the word "believe" and not "think"'?

As a doctor, it is likely that at some stage in our career we will be involved in a legal case. Hopefully not directly, but there is tremendous wealth in the sports industry, and some legal teams now specialise in sports litigation cases. I worry when I hear about junior doctors covering professional football matches. I hope they are aware of the potential implications on their future careers if something were to go wrong. My advice is for them to thoroughly check with indemnity providers about all the components of the role and ensure that they have not been left exposed in any way. Court cases are public. Observing a medical negligence claim as a learning process is something I wish I had done earlier in my career.

Tips for Success

Working in SEM can be isolating in some instances. I believe it is vital for young consultants to have mentors and safe platforms to discuss cases, concerns or any of the things that stop you from drifting off at night.

Junior doctors often ask how to get into sports medicine, and many have an interest in football. What they possibly overlook is that our speciality consists of sport *and* exercise medicine. I encourage them to invest their time in public health, whether in schools or community-based events. Encouraging the next generation of SEM doctors to push and advocate for physical activity gives our message greater outreach and helps protect future generations.

Our health systems are suffering greatly under the demands of physical inactivity, and I would love to see more public health jobs developing to help combat this. In the meantime, we must continue to promote and push physical activity to encourage patients and communities to make changes. We should act as role models to society and demonstrate all the ways that we are active in our daily lives and with our families. Working alongside successful athletes can be thrilling. But the thrill of witnessing the achievements of amateur athletes, or those who make changes from being physically inactive, is profound. Exercise is medicine. This is a fact. Simple, powerful and true. As Johann Wolfgang von Goethe eloquently said, 'Whatever you dream you can do, begin it. Boldness has genius, power, and magic in it. Begin it now'.

Setbacks, Success, Personal Stories and Reflections – Jacopo Mattaini

Introduction

Renzo Piano, one of the most successful and internationally recognised Italian architects, once said, 'The journey is discovering, it is life. Younger generations should move away from Italy, as long as they come back'.

In that interview, Renzo was pushing young architects to new experiences abroad not only for professional growth but also to make them realise how lucky they are to live in Italy and to further appreciate the amazing art and building culture of their and my country.

At the time of this interview, I was at the very beginning of my career as a physio, completely opposite from a discipline such as architecture, but those words, his vision and the values he wanted to transmit really struck me. I felt he was speaking to me, like there were no differences at all between his job and my field, sports medicine. Still today, I resemble his thoughts, and I bet many of you are inspired by those words like I was. Well, if you are, here is the good news: physiotherapy has no boundaries, the human body is absolutely the same in every corner of this planet and our profession has reasons to exist in all those corners. Potentially any of you can collect work experience in other countries to enrich your clinical skills and, most importantly, your persona.

Fortune Favours the Brave

So far, my journey as a physiotherapist is remarkably linked to travel, exploration and personal growth. Everything started in 2009; after my bachelor's degree in Milan, I moved to Fort Lauderdale, Florida, where I could continue studying physiotherapy through an athletic scholarship. I played soccer in the NCAA for my university, and they paid for my studies for the doctor of physical therapy program. Pretty cool, eh? Yes, I admit it, such a lucky catch! Many things had to align for me to start that adventure, but you know what they say: fortune favours the brave. It happened because I wanted it, because I was inspired and I really believed I could achieve that goal of mine: to live abroad at least once in my life. That first experience really forged me, and after completing 2 years of studies in the United States, something clicked: I wanted more; I wanted to have other experiences outside Italy, this time practising. So after a brief working period back home (still in a different city, to fulfil my hunger for change), I ended up moving again. In 2016 I moved to London and then in 2019 to New York, where I still live.

The past 13 years have gone so quickly, and they have been incredible: the number of people, cultures, lifestyles and values I crossed paths with are countless. I can proudly say that I have worked and treated patients from all six populated continents.

Now, stop for one second and imagine a broader picture for yourself. As physiotherapists, we can really diversify in many work positions: we can choose between clinical work, teaching and research; we can work in public health or privately; we can specialise in orthopaedic or neurologic rehabilitation, for example; we can focus on sports medicine or more general population; we can target more specific clients such athletes, dancers, musicians or art performers. It does not matter if you are still studying, if you just started a new or even your first job or if you have been working for many years, there are always opportunities somewhere, even more if you are willing to move to other cities or outside your own country.

Needs Must

In my case, the first time I decided to move was during my studies: the main reason was the insufficiency of my courses in Italy and the sensation that I needed something more to educate and prepare myself for the job world out there. I was in my third and last year of physiotherapy degree in Italy, finishing up my clinical internships and writing my final thesis. There were so many holes in my education and the idea that in a few months I would have been on my own with patients, leading their rehabilitation, was really frightening.

I was not ready at all, and honestly, it felt like I was a bit responsible, and I kept asking myself: 'Am I lazy? Should I have studied more? Why am I feeling so unprepared?' I wanted to grow in orthopaedic rehabilitation and, being an athlete myself, to explore the sports medicine world – an educational field where I felt that my university failed me.

Those words from Renzo Piano really pushed me to take an extra step, getting out of my comfort zone and considering an experience abroad. That opportunity in Florida was a pure blessing and one of the best things that ever happened to me. The infrastructure, the professors and the course structures really elevated the clinical aspect of my learning journey to a world-class level. However, what really enriched me as an individual was doing all that away from home, learning from new cultures, meeting new people and of course living my daily life in a language that, at that time, I had only studied a few hours per week at school.

For the first time I realised the importance of communication in a multidisciplinary environment, from choosing the right words for my papers and conversations with professors to my calls to teammates during a soccer match (it took me ages to understand common football tactical calls like 'Right/left shoulder!' to indicate an opponent nearby you or 'Squeeze!' to close up the opponent team in the midfield). The international community was so big that I really learnt the meaning of respect, diversity, integration and sharing, values that I embrace every day with my patients.

That experience enriched me with the clinical and soft skills that are needed to succeed as a physiotherapist. It served to fuel my ambition to become a consistently better version of myself. I encountered situations where I was pushed out of my comfort zone, turning the experience into a fantastic growth opportunity.

A few years later, when in London I started supervising students from other countries, I realised how education was a catalyst to modelling, shifting and progressing to a new status. I learnt about different degree structures, some over 4, 5 or even 7 years: a better situation compared to my 3 years as an undergraduate. I was often impressed by their knowledge and clinical reasoning; they were way ahead compared to the younger version of myself right after Italian college. That's why, looking back, I truly believe that moving abroad was the best choice I have ever made, and I would do it again and again.

Now, 13 years later, I also see that those same degrees offered in my country have now improved massively and that the educational programs are levelling up with the international scene.

Step Outside Your Comfort Zone

Regarding continuing education, maybe nowadays it is not that necessary to move abroad for better courses: many countries are offering valuable and high-level master's and doctoral degrees that can satisfy your desires and shape your professional career. However, if any of you are feeling unprepared in terms of education, or just simply looking to continue studying and live a nice life, nothing will enrich you as much as pushing yourself out of your comfort zone and studying in another country.

The second and third times I moved abroad were job related. Since I enjoyed my first experience, it was an easier decision for myself. As you can imagine, and probably some of you can also relate to, the key elements that pushed me were financial aspects, working stability and better prospects.

What It Means to Travel

Migration is the story of humankind, and no matter what, we are always looking for better solutions for ourselves and our families. As physiotherapists, if we are not satisfied with the current situation or looking for new experience, we can ride the same wave and look for a better chance away from home. However, nothing comes free and without obstacles: language examination and national exams for foreign licences are the toughest barriers you might encounter in your process. I will tell you a secret: in my first attempt at my exam for the US licence, I failed! Despite this initial frustration, I kept working on it and eventually passed. In terms of requirements, some countries are tougher than others, with more difficult exams and complex rules. Failure should be considered a plausible part of the process.

As Winston Churchill once said, 'Success is stumbling from failure to failure with no loss of enthusiasm'. Therefore, despite the results, learn how to look at these tests as the first opportunities to be a better version of yourself: from improving a foreign language to reviewing the clinical concepts and latest evidence in literature; these are all elements that will make you a better clinician.

Working abroad has been great. The things I have enjoyed the most are the multicultural aspects – sharing the workspace with colleagues and patients from other countries and backgrounds. There are no schools or degrees that can truly prepare you and help you grow like these experiences.

Learning Within Novel Structures

All the healthcare professionals, while having different roles and responsibilities across different countries, are all aiming to provide the best care for the person in front of you. For example, in the UK I have studied and included in my treatment bag dry needling, a technique which is not permitted in Italy or in the state of New York. In the US, athletic trainers (ATs) can use manual treatment approaches or hands-on modalities with athletes, while ATs in Italy can only prescribe exercise and plan the strength and conditioning programmes with their clients. During sports events, doctors in Italy are usually the ones performing emergency response, while in the US that practice belongs to ATs and an array of first responders. What I want to say is that, while working within the specified constraints, we should always base treatment for our patients on scientific literature and what evidence notes as best practice.

Moving countries caused me to adapt my practice as a physiotherapist, and as a result it enriched my bag of skills and improved my treatment approaches. As a clinician, I learnt to treat my patients using what I had available. Multidisciplinary teams in different settings may have alternative structures, with the same professionals in different countries sometimes performing tasks in altered ways. Therefore, my connection to others within these interdisciplinary teams was paramount: sharing my role, learning from others and further living and developing my values such as communication, respect, trust and transparency.

Final Remarks

In conclusion, I believe that, like you, I have been striving for a long time. My career required me to look outside typical geographical and institutional borders and consider experiences away from home. I am not and do not want to sound like a person who has a disdain for their own country. What strikes me is that the more I experience life abroad, the more I appreciate life and the professionals in my home country. I never detached completely from my Italian colleagues and students: I saw the movement growing, with physios who remained home and others who, like me, had an experience abroad, coming together and pushing our professional ceilings to new heights.

This is something that really makes me proud. Maybe one day I will go back home and practise sports medicine in Italy, because after 13 years I am even more convinced that Renzo Piano was absolutely right!

Setbacks, Success, Personal Stories and Reflections – Carl Gombrich

Introduction

'This chapter looks at the intersection between interdisciplinary practice and the gaining of soft skills. I will argue that more exposure to interdisciplinarity will help physiotherapists in soft skills development.'

I wrote this introductory paragraph after discussing my 'story' contribution to this volume with one of the editors, David Clancy. As usual with a book chapter, there had been a few false starts and dead-ends before it became obvious, through my experiences in interdisciplinary education, that one gain from all kinds of interdisciplinary learning and working is the acquiring of soft skills. David had written to me that he saw 'listening, asking better questions, being curious' and 'empathy' as key soft skills for physiotherapists, and there was plenty of overlap here with what I knew had surfaced as key skills for good interdisciplinary working (Becerra, 2021; Labzina *et al.*, 2019).

Hence the intro.

What Does AI Say?

But then, because it's hard to resist right now, I typed into ChatGPT, 'What is the relationship between interdisciplinarity and soft skills?', and I got this:

'Interdisciplinary practice involves the integration of knowledge and methods from different disciplines to address complex problems. Soft skills, on the other hand, refer to personal attributes and social abilities that enable individuals to interact effectively with others and perform well in a team-based setting.'

'Interdisciplinary practice requires individuals to have strong soft skills such as communication, collaboration, empathy, adaptability, and critical thinking. When working in interdisciplinary teams, individuals need to be able to communicate effectively with team members from different backgrounds, understand and appreciate diverse perspectives, and be willing to adapt their approach to accommodate different ways of thinking.'

'Furthermore, interdisciplinary practice often involves working in complex and dynamic environments, where problem-solving requires the ability to think critically, creatively, and independently. Soft skills such as adaptability, emotional intelligence, and resilience, are essential for individuals to be successful in such environments.'

'In summary, interdisciplinary practice and soft skills are closely related, as individuals who possess strong soft skills are better equipped to work effectively in interdisciplinary teams and contribute to solving complex problems.'

This is pretty good! And I really didn't have to think about the prompt. I just typed in my 'essay question' and there's the answer. I urge you to read it again as it's dense and covers a lot of ground. It is similar to how I would answer the question myself and aligned with, for example, the explanation provided in Becerra (2021). To complete what ChatGPT has offered us, it doesn't look like there's much to do other than flesh things out and provide some evidence and some references. And maybe that's OK. If the new AI can suggest things we agree with, and then if the 'chain of authority' for whatever we rest our knowledge claims on can be traced back to credible sources, good evidence and/or the originator of the idea, then what else could we ask for in terms of reliable knowledge?

Scene Setting

So, I'm going to run with this. But let's slow the pace down. We need to back up a bit. Explain how we got here. Explain how and why I'm writing this chapter. Context and credibility, in other words.

But before even this, a note on the style of this chapter. You may be thinking it's a bit informal. Perhaps it doesn't appear suitably 'academic'. This is deliberate. My colleague at the London Interdisciplinary School, James Carney, himself an expert in AI and large language models (LLMs) that are dominating the current discussion, says: 'We are going to see a return to much more personal styles of academic writing now that AI has mastered the bland, neutral approach'. I take this seriously. Because how would you know if this whole chapter wasn't written by AI, using a series of prompts, unless there were personal touches that you could check? And so long as the references in a piece of writing can be backed up (something AI is currently not great at) then feigning a more 'neutral' or 'objective' style may come to appear as something of an exercise in 'smoke and mirrors', which, in fact, it always was.

Interdisciplinarity, the Allied Medical Professions and Me

I believe in the power and relevance of interdisciplinary education for most graduate jobs in today's knowledge and digital economy (Gombrich, 2016). The world is changing fast (Rosa, 2015) and the connection between standard academic disciplines and most graduate jobs is almost completely broken (ISE, 2020). I have also seen the essential contributions of various forms of interdisciplinary practice (Ecological Brain, 2023; ITRC, 2020). For the past 13 years, I have been involved in leading the design of programmes and institutions that deliver interdisciplinary education and I've had the privilege and pleasure of seeing the benefits that such a way of learning has for thousands of students. Yet, despite being passionate about interdisciplinarity, and despite having lots of evidence about how and why it can work, there are still times when it is hard to explain what I do, and why I think it's important. And often the hardest group of people for me to explain this to are medics and allied professionals such as dentists or, indeed, physiotherapists.

Why is this? Well, partly it is because medicine and the allied professions remain highly credentialed, with licences to practise protected by law, and registers of licensed practitioners kept, in the case of physiotherapists, by the Health and Care Professions Council. This 'top-down' approach then informs everything from codes of conduct to university syllabi and exams, to continuing professional development. In many ways this is a good thing! The original Hippocratic oath, the basis of much medical ethics in Western medicine, has more than one injunction to 'do no harm.' Without tight regulation and oversight, it would be much easier for bad actors to enter the system and cause harm to their patients.

However, this tightly controlled, hierarchical system also has drawbacks. Firstly, there are the well-documented cases of medical errors and poor decision-making, and the difficulties in such hierarchical cultures of speaking up in order to reduce errors (Epstein, 2019; Syed, 2015). Then there is the question of how a tightly controlled and regulated practice can allow for innovation. The graduates from the programmes I am involved in work in some of the hundreds of new, interdisciplinary sectors springing up in our knowledge and digital economies: AI and Law, Sustainable Energy, Fintech, Cybersecurity, Sustainable Food Systems, Design Thinking, Data Visualisation and so on. My discussions with medics and the like of these new and exciting areas of graduate employment are generally met with blank stares. Where is the time and headspace to collaborate in new and innovative ways if your education requires you to progress on a path that is completely mapped out in advance and required to hit many predetermined milestones along the way? The idea of a more interdisciplinary approach to education seems alien to many of these professionals as it plays little part in their working lives.

The State of Play

However, there are signs that the allied professions may be open to change. For example, a recent paper shows recognition of a type of 'knowledge gap' in physiotherapy training (Schwab *et al.*, 2023). The authors argue that physiotherapists need wider, more interdisciplinary training (including exposure to nonmedical fields) in order to assist 'within [the] individual [patient's] unique environmental and social realities', and that physiotherapists would be advantaged by being able to 'leverage knowledge and methods in another scientific discipline'. Parallel to this recognition of more *intellectual* knowledge gaps, Clancy (2023) writes, 'we [physiotherapists] are not educated [in soft skills] in third level institutions at all, nor in clinical placements or postgraduate grading'.

If the ChatGPT response is correct (more on that in a moment), there is an excellent opportunity for synergy here: more interdisciplinary learning, required by physiotherapists to be better practitioners in a fast-changing world, will also help deliver to them the soft skills missing from their training.

Learning Soft Skills From Being More Interdisciplinary

Returning to our ChatGPT response, we see it picks out the following soft skills: 'communication, collaboration [teamwork], empathy, adaptability, and critical thinking'. In case we have any reason to doubt these choices, this is a good subsection of a list from a well-known jobs and HR website (Workable, 2023).

Let's take these one by one and show that such skills are also required in interdisciplinary contexts. (We omit 'critical thinking' here for reasons of space and because it is a less obviously 'human-centred' soft skill.) For example, Gabriele Bammer, in her series of blogs on interdisciplinary practice, says that the key to solving complex interdisciplinary problems with stakeholders is 'consultation, involvement, collaboration … being able to listen … in order to understand … perspectives, concerns' (Bammer, 2021). In this quote we see the need for good communication and collaboration.

Empathy, in the list above and in Clancy's list of key soft skills, is often associated with perspective-taking (Neuroscience News, 2020), and perspective-taking is a key part of successful interdisciplinary learning (Gombrich & Hogan, 2017). Empathy is perhaps unusually difficult to build in some academic contexts (Gombrich, 2013). This is because academic disciplines can encourage strong worldviews (Becher & Trowler, 2001), which then make types of perspective-taking difficult. For example, academics from the humanities or social sciences may think all knowledge is 'socially constructed' and therefore relative to the community in which it sits, whereas scientists or engineers may be wedded to the idea of objective facts that are independent of any cultural context. When working in an interdisciplinary team, say on a project related to sustainability, an academic more concerned with social justice and the possible effects of climate change on poorer communities may be challenged by another academic who regards the science as neutral and does not wish to bring politics into the discussion (and vice versa). This difference may manifest in 'lack of appreciation for the other disciplines' and an 'uncompromising and defensive disciplinary stance' (Gyampoh, 2018). Successful interdisciplinary work will thus involve overcoming these negative positions through challenging oneself to be better at intellectual perspective-taking, thus increasing empathy with colleagues. We can't know for sure whether this 'high-level' intellectual perspective-taking can help with wider challenges of empathy, but it seems likely that if you are able to learn to empathise with world views radically different to your own, then empathising with others in more everyday matters will be easier.

Just as we can posit a relationship between academic empathy and everyday empathy, we can also posit a relationship between 'epistemic adaptability' (Horn *et al.*, 2022) and the adaptability widely listed as a key soft skill. Epistemic adaptability requires 'accommodating behaviour' and 'engaging with others' knowledge.' As with the example of empathy above, it seems likely that if you are adaptable in this epistemic way, other types of adaptability will come more easily.

Concluding Thoughts

My hunch was that there was a good intersection between learning soft skills and learning and working in interdisciplinary contexts. This was corroborated by what I thought was an excellent first response from ChatGPT. Why should you believe this is a good answer? I argue that that ultimately depends on what you think of my credibility in this space, and the authenticity of the experiences and references to other work that I can provide. I then noted that medicine and the allied professions, including physiotherapy, still struggle – for several reasons – to engage widely with interdisciplinarity. But there are signs of change. Examples were given of when interdisciplinarity has taught – or at least fostered – better communication, collaboration, perspective-taking (empathy) and adaptability, which are widely acknowledged as core soft skills. It would therefore be of value for physiotherapists to spend part of their training in interdisciplinary learning and practice to acquire these skills.

ChatGPT has helped me in this chapter. Does it have soft skills? Maybe some, but most soft skills will, for the foreseeable future, be about human-to-human interactions – far harder to master than what AI has so far achieved. Physiotherapists who understand this and engage in the discussion about and learning of soft skills are likely to be able to survive much of the oncoming AI revolution.

References

Bammer, G. (2021). Stakeholder engagement primer: 7. Listening and dialogue. *Integration and Implementation Insights*. Available at https://i2insights.org/.

Becerra, M. (2021). The need for interdisciplinarity in higher education. *Forbes*. Available at https://www.forbes.com/.

Becher, T., & Trowler, P. (2001). *Academic tribes and territories*. Berkshire: Open University Press.

Clancy, D. (2023). Email to Carl Gombrich, 17 May.

Ecological Brain. (2023). Available at http://www.ecologicalbrain.org.

Epstein, D. (2019). *Range: Why generalists triumph in a specialized world.* Available at https://davidepstein.com/.

Gombrich, C. (2013). Academic empathy. Available at http://www.carlgombrich.org/.

Gombrich, C. (2016). *Polymathy, new generalism, and the future of work: A little theory and some practice from UCL's arts and sciences degree.* SpringerLink. Available at https://link.springer.com/.

Gombrich, C., & Hogan, P. (2017). Interdisciplinarity and the student voice. In *The Oxford handbook of interdisciplinarity.* Available at https://academic.oup.com/.

Gyampoh, B. A. (2018). The challenges of interdisciplinarity: Insights from a research programme on climate change. Ecosystem Services for Poverty Alleviation. Available at https://www.espa.ac.uk/news-blogs/blog/challenges-interdisciplinarity-insights-research-programme-climate-change. Accessed 12 March 2024.

Horn, R., Urian, L., & Zweekhorst, M. (2022). *Epistemic stability and epistemic adaptability: Interdisciplinary knowledge integration competencies for complex sustainability issues.* SpringerLink. Available at https://link.springer.com/.

ISE. (2020). *University evolution.* London Interdisciplinary School. Available at https://www.lis.ac.uk/.

ITRC. (2020). Lena Fuldauer awarded 1st prize in the Allianz Climate Risk Research Award. Available at https://www.itrc.org.uk/.

Labzina, P., Dobrova, V., Menshenina, S., & Ageenko, N. (2019). Forming a new quality of interdisciplinary education as a way to overcome the crisis phenomena in the development of modern society. In *Proceedings of the 2018 International Conference on Computer Science and Information Systems (CSIS'18).* Atlantis Press. https://doi.org/10.2991/csis-18.2019.69.

Neuroscience News. (2020). Empathy and perspective taking: How social skills are built. Available at https://neurosciencenews.com/.

Rosa, H. (2015). *Social acceleration: A new theory of modernity.* New York, NY: Columbia University Press.

Schwab, S. M., Andrade, A. D., Seibt, A. C., Zech, A., Karayannis, N. V., Meurer, A., … Beattie, P. (2023). Narrowing the physiotherapy knowledge-practice gap: Faculty training beyond the health sciences. *Journal of Interprofessional Care, 37*(1), 127–136. https://doi.org/10.1080/13561820.2022.2028625.

Syed, M. (2015). *Black box thinking: The surprising truth about success.* London: John Murray Press.

Workable. (2023). What are soft skills? Top 15 soft skills examples. Available at https://www.workable.com/.

CLOSING REMARKS – PUTTING IT ALL TOGETHER

Ciaran Dunne ▪ David Clancy

'Human skills required to be a better human.'

Simon Sinek, inspirational speaker and author of *Start With Why* and *The Infinite Game*. (He identifies a pattern in great leaders and organisations in terms of their ability to communicate … that there are countless metrics to measure performance, but few to measure trust properly. For Sinek, and us, the authors, the soft skills are essential.)

Final Words

Thank you for being here. You could have chosen to do many things right now, but instead you chose to be here reading our book. You chose the path of learning, from others – and, from yourself. You were curious. You are the embodiment of a 'Learning Physiotherapist'.

It is often said that the path to greatness is along with others. Picking up this book to learn from others signals that you will experience growth throughout your career.

In this closing chapter, we discuss a few more ideas for you to reflect on, and our final thoughts on the lessons and insights in this book. We do hope you have found *Essential Skills for Physiotherapists* a revolutionary and transformative textbook for your life, not just your career.

Relational Performance

Small talk matters. It often builds meaningful connections. Dr. Brené Brown once proclaimed, 'I define connection as the energy that exists between people when they feel seen, heard and valued; when they can give and receive without judgement; and when they derive sustenance and strength from the relationship' (Brown, 2019). How we interact with each other matters. How well we get along matters.

Today there is much uncertainty around cohesion, collaboration, trust and other social elements that build connections and improve relationships. Important questions are arising – How can we improve communication here? How can we make feedback a normal behaviour? How do we build our team for sustained success? Wellbeing and performance are inextricably linked in our opinion, and social wellbeing needs some time in the light now. For us, social wellbeing means relational performance (RP), which we define as 'thriving and achieving through teamwork'.

RP is an evidence-based, scientifically informed framework (developed by Hauora Ltd., inspired by case studies at the intersection of business and professional sport, and publications such as *Harvard Business Review* and McKinsey & Company) that operates at three levels, namely individual, team and organisational; it is comprised of four domains: boldness, cohesion, communication and psychological safety. The concept transcends anything learned in clinical academia, delving into the essential skills. The framework is best represented as a wheel with 4 domains and 16 components (refer to the following image).

Each domain houses the key ingredients to becoming a better version of yourself as you interact with your own mind and the world around you (for definitions, see the table).

Bringing It Together

This book represents what we believe is the primary reason for getting ahead in your personal and professional life – the soft skills, embedded within the RP framework. RP encapsulates what

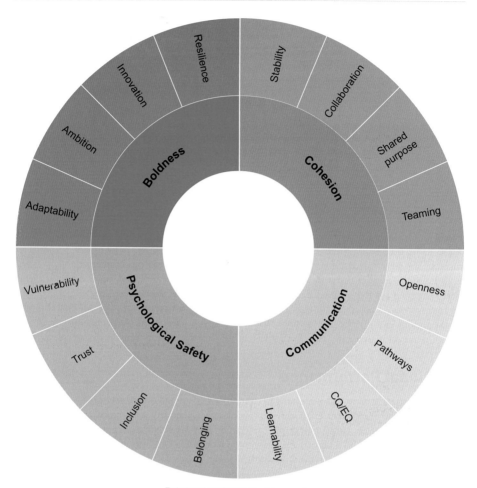

Relational performance framework.

it takes to strive and thrive, individually and together. We must connect well with not only our-selves but with one another. By doing this we provide the platform for sustained performance and growth as we aim for new heights in our careers.

Lean In – Boldness

The great American poet Robert Frost said, 'freedom lies in being bold', and how right he was (Hamburger, 1952, p. 169). To achieve all you are capable of (think of your ambition), you must be courageous, take risks and experience failures. The freedom that you earn from this is not a lack of responsibility but more a wealth of life.

We must step outside the comfort zone, be adaptable like a limber pine facing an avalanche, and be resilient – that age-old analogy, to get back on the horse. Understanding trends, worldviews and what novel approaches you can adopt speaks to an innovative mindset, a potentially huge competitive advantage in our profession.

Relational Performance Definitions

Domain	Component	Definition
Cohesion 'Working with unity and commitment towards a common goal'	Stability	Working with the same people for a sustained time frame
	Collaboration	Working well with others to achieve a shared outcome
	Shared purpose	Embracing and pursuing a common objective
	Teaming	Collaborating and coordinating to get important things done
Communication 'Exchanging information and ideas efficiently and effectively'	Pathways	Having multiple means to exchange information
	EQ/CQ	Possessing high emotional and cultural capabilities
	Learnability	Becoming familiar with new content with ease and speed
	Openness	Being receptive to new ideas, opinions or arguments
Psychological Safety 'Sharing ideas, questions, or concerns without interpersonal fear'	Belonging	Feeling accepted and valued
	Inclusion	Respecting everyone's needs, perspectives and potential
	Trust	Being accountable to and supportive of each other
	Vulnerability	Willingness to express genuine thoughts and feelings
Boldness 'Thinking and acting beyond existing organisational limits'	Adaptability	Adjusting to different conditions or circumstances
	Ambition	Strongly desiring a goal or objective
	Innovation	Generating new ideas, concepts, things, etc.
	Resilience	Overcoming unexpected change or adversity

1 + 1 = 3 – Cohesion

Cohesion relates to a collective commitment to a common goal that truly drives progress and achievement. Without cohesion, it is difficult to achieve sustainability, stability and progress. When we work in a clinic, as part of a sports team or in a large hospital or trust, we are constantly surrounded by or interacting with people. Even a sole trader or lone worker will interact with others via email communication, social media, clinical work or even regulatory bodies.

Collaboration is the key to all teamwork, but when the team is ever changing, we need to have the skill of teaming allowing us to work with new people and get up to speed on the fly – consider the critical outreach team in a large hospital as an example.

Within teams a certain level of stability is vital. It allows for familiarisation with others and their traits, personalities and habits. To build this we must work with people who we can be ourselves with; we must understand each other. To work as an even more high-performing unit we must possess a shared purpose. Think for a moment about the famous, all-conquering New Zealand All Blacks rugby team – their culture and behaviours on and off the pitch have been well documented. They emphasise humility, hard work and respect for their opponents, and they use their shared purpose to motivate themselves and stay focused on their goals. They 'sweep the sheds', as James Kerr wrote in *Legacy* (Kerr, 2013). A winning formula.

Being Able to Be You – Psychological Safety

Challenge is a positive, in almost any sense. In our careers it presents the obstacles we must over-come to upskill and become better, for example, telling a client about their diagnosis. In life it is part of the evolutionary system, such as reducing morbidity risk as we grow old. Finally in our own minds, challenge often comes from within, and it is our ability to share and make sense of these challenges that will equate to how well we ultimately overcome them.

Where challenge presents itself, we must face it with a certain vulnerability. This does not mean shying away or succumbing to the adversity faced. Quite the opposite. It means leaning into discomfort with an honest view of self, others and the situation. This is psychological safety – the ability to speak up or challenge without fear of retribution.

It is a concept that is spoken about in groups, organisations and teams; however, it also exists within us. We must challenge unhelpful thoughts, beliefs and biases each day to get to the best decisions in life. Inclusion, and that sense of feeling part of something, belonging, is critical for our wellbeing ... for that of being accepted, trusted and valued, ingredients for self and group performance.

The Bridge Between – Communication

George Bernard Shaw, the famed Irish playwright, once said, 'The single biggest problem in com-munication is the illusion that it has taken place' (Caroselli, 2000). As physiotherapists commu-nication is the cornerstone of how we assess, treat, understand and support our clients. It is a skill that we must train and constantly review.

The RP framework highlights four components that, once enhanced, will exponentially improve our ability to connect with others using our communication. Forging pathways such as our listening abilities, our use of language and our body language make tangible differences. Having high levels of cultural and emotional intelligence will breed life into our relationships. It provides the dials we must manipulate to align with different situations and people around us. Learnability, how quickly and with how much ease we can absorb, process and take on new information, is worth upskilling in, along with openness – the level of receptivity we give to new ideas, opinions or arguments.

It is no secret that many courses in physiotherapy highlight and aim to train communication and its many styles and approaches; however, understanding the above components, along with the insights in Chapter 4, can help catapult us to new heights!

Speaking and Writing – The Game Changers

For us, self-education and constant training in public speaking and writing has been massively influential in our careers. The ability to clearly articulate your thoughts, feelings and stories using your voice is a skill that all practitioners must study and practice. It can seem daunting at first, scary even, but it is a competitive advantage. Consider investing in courses to improve the art of oral communication; it is critical for influence and persuasion, negotiation, creating buy-in, moti-vation and bringing people together. Messy or poorly delivered communication can make any situation worse – think about delivering information to a patient, presenting a topic at a confer-ence or speaking with a peer even.

Look for opportunities. Seek them. Seminars and forums. A poster presentation. A podcast interview. Anything that tests your speaking skills (body language, tone of voice, etc.). Study the masters, from in the profession and outside the profession. Look at world-renowned orators like Ed Mylett (motivational speaker and author of *The Power of One More*), Rian Doris (CEO of the Flow Research Collective), Robin Sharma (author of *The 5 AM Club*), Les Brown (dynamic, globally recognised speaker), Tony Robbins (author of *Awaken the Giant Within*) and Laura Gassner Otting (author of *Limitless*), for example. What is it about them that stands out? The Heath Brothers (Chip and Dan) are worth exploring too!

The Heath Brothers have a formula (acronym even!) for six qualities of sticky ideas, which one could use when speaking (Heath & Heath, 2007).

SUCCESs:

- Simple – a succinct message
- Unexpected – leveraging surprise and intrigue as assets
- Concrete – ensuring your idea is grounded and relatable
- Credible – giving the audience proof by way of statistics, testimonies or examples
- Emotional – triggering a response of joy, sadness or fun
- Stories – storytelling helps make information stay in our memory

Now, let's pivot to writing.

Can you fight the resistance that faces you with a blank page? Sit with it and write – be the professional, as Steven Pressfield unpacks in *The War of Art* (Pressfield, 2002). Writing forces you to pay attention and helps you understand what you believe. Writing is not just an activity, but a way of seeing the world. It is about living a richer, more fulfilling life and attracting the people you want to share it with, as online writing guru and host of 'Write of Passage' David Perell puts it.

Digital content creator and futurist Dan Koe talks about how writing implies understanding and learning of inputs … and that it helps capture attention and persuade – and even create significant revenue streams. Another titan of writing, and someone who has influenced us, David Hieatt, Co-Founder of Hiut Denim Co. and The Do Lectures, is active in building influential global brands and helping people become copywriters and keyboard CEOs. For us, writing plays a big role in generating traffic to our websites and courses – growth opportunities in essence. It is the marketing and sales medium we need to get competent at, and confident with. Hieatt has models in his email writing such as hook, story and close – and often builds SAME into his writing:

- Story
- Analogy
- Metaphor
- Example

This can help make your writing more memorable and relatable. Try it! It works for emails, blogs, articles … book chapters even. Study the 'voice' and tone you want to use when writing – do you want the reader to absorb your material in a playful way, a professional way, casual or engaging?

Steven Kotler, acclaimed author and peak performance expert, speaks about using somatic address when writing. Can you elicit an emotional response in the reader? There is a way to trigger the release of certain neurochemicals, by choice of words, style of writing and other tools of the art to spark a feeling.

If you want to change your game, upskill and constantly deliver in speaking and writing. Create and 'just do it'. Nike got it right.

A Journey of Growth

Embarking on the path to becoming a highly successful and compassionate physiotherapist possesses many similarities to becoming a proficient and capable accountant, mechanic, salesperson or nurse, for example. It is our ability to nurture a grounded and authentic sense of purpose and values, hone effective communication skills, have willpower and foster habits that propel us towards sustained peak performance. We get ahead of those around us by seeking mentorship, being clear on goals, maintaining discipline and motivation and perhaps even building a personal brand.

Your career must be an adventure filled with immense personal and professional growth. Drawing insights from distinguished thought leaders, this book, with focal areas around wellbeing, working with others, career mapping and high performance, is designed to empower you by arming you with the essential tools to navigate the ever-evolving landscape of a career in physiotherapy.

Put On Your Own Mask First!

Physiotherapists are expanding their lens and exploring what they do, why they do it and how they can align these two. In the first section of this book, we lay the foundations of becoming an accomplished professional, by looking after yourself first. By identifying your personal values and aligning them with your purpose, we are ensuring that during difficult times or when facing hard decisions, we know we act and proceed in a manner that is at peace with our character and who we are deep down.

When we do not act in accordance with this truth, we put ourselves at risk of burnout, heightened anxiety and illness, conditions that are not uncommon for physiotherapists to experience in clinics, hospitals or sports/healthcare organisations.

Managing personal wellbeing is a necessity. Burnout is the extreme stage – it is when it is too late, and we need drastic or immediate intervention. Proactively looking after wellbeing – physically, mentally and socially – is vital for us all. Use the first section of this book as an exploration of what drives us, what is important to you and habit formation – and to know how this can become fuel to your fire. Furthermore, we must acknowledge the necessity of striking a balance between personal wellbeing and professional growth, as this equilibrium ensures enduring success and resilience in this demanding yet rewarding field.

Connecting and Working With Others

Who do you admire? Consider this for a moment. What is it about them? Why do you feel this way towards them?

Humans are considered the apex mammal because of our ability to connect, integrate and build tribes with others. We value social connectedness as an imperative in our journey towards fulfilment and satisfaction. Understanding ourselves is where you start, but the next step relates to our ability to understand and connect with others. Hunt for opportunities to connect and collaborate, to build something special with others … to learn from each other. This can take you to the next level. As Steven Kotler says, understand that curiosity can lead to passion, purpose, focused attention and flow – peak performance (Kotler, 2014). Revisit chapters in this book on communication, mentorship and working with others cohesively to truly become a part of your tribe.

Career Mapping

The success of your career can come down to the number of difficult conversations you are willing to have, with you and others. Our ability to face challenges and to struggle not only helps us achieve more, but it also makes us stronger. Tenacity and persistence are vital – as the San Antonio Spurs of the NBA proclaim, 'Keep pounding the rock'.

We learn about treating the whole person in front of us, not the injury, ailment or disease. We promote holistic pathways to recovery for our clients, and we provide a comprehensive roadmap for their journey. Yet too often we overlook our career roadmap. Our very own journey must focus on curiosity, continuous learning, setting goals and, maybe, building a personal brand (Chapter 9 is a must-read!). The fascinating insights here illuminate the value of strategic planning and adaptability in the ever-evolving field of physiotherapy.

Achieving High Performance

What makes high performers tick? What a valuable question. Success leaves clues. As Dwayne 'The Rock' Johnson often says, 'focus and keep your eyes on the prize'; there is so much to be said for being intentional with where you place your attention. We must remember that. You will not have to look far for inspiration – it is present each day, and as Oliver Burkeman (2022) wrote, we live for roughly 4000 weeks … so our time here is limited. Use this precious resource wisely and think about what you say yes to, and what you say no to. Be where your feet are.

Through small and large feats, we see humans win, lose, overcome and sustain excellence. Find your inspiration – hopefully it lies within the pages of this book – and embody the lessons there every day. Constantly reread the sections on life/work alignment, dealing with stress, mental fitness and leading yourself and others with purpose to achieve what is true high performance. The score will take care of itself (Walsh, 2010).

Mastery Inspired by Mentors

What an inspiration it is to hear stories, successes and failures from some of the best physiotherapists in the world. We can learn a lot from examining the careers of people who have walked the path before us – echoes of the seminal book *Mastery* by Robert Greene (2012).

Chapter 14 details the paths taken by industry and thought leaders, including the ups and downs, the achievements, insights, setbacks and origin stories. These journeys serve as a testament to the transformative power of embracing soft skills.

Learn and Give Back

One of the most powerful ways to grow is to help others. It is said that our relative chances of being on this earth are approximately 0.000000000025% or 1 in 4 trillion (Robbins, 2011). Let that sink in for a moment. These are staggering numbers, but taken within the correct perspective, they are a reminder of how fortunate we are – and how precious life and education is.

No matter what adversity we face each day – and do understand, we are all faced with something – there is always someone who we can support or help. At 'The Learning Physiotherapist' we continuously remind ourselves of this. We strive to support those who have not been as fortunate as us or who don't have the opportunities or resources we do. And this is vital. It has also supported medical research and charities for Down syndrome, breast cancer, prostate cancer, irritable bowel syndrome (IBS) and mental health.

A philosophy has fuelled the mission and purpose of our group from the very start. If there is one wish we have from your reading of this book, it is for you to get better … but when you do, to also please reach out and bring someone else up with you. Support those around you and those who need it.

As we have said from day one, 'Learn and Give Back'.

Final Thoughts

All the authors here are hoping to inspire physiotherapists to unlock their potential by embracing a holistic approach to personal and professional development. By integrating the essential soft skills, principles and practices filled within these pages, you will be poised to tackle the challenges and take the opportunities that await, resulting in fulfilling and influential careers in physiotherapy.

Overall, this book aims to be your companion on your journey in your career and in your life. There is plenty of science, anecdotal references, and captivating stories here, from an eclectic and cognitively diverse group. The lessons and gold within are not siloed to your career as a physiotherapist – but can enhance your experience in all aspects of living. Use this book as a tool. Bring it with you. Reflect on it. Write about it; share your thoughts on it. Ultimately, the heights you reach in your career often reflect how well you learn and execute the soft skills that make all the difference.

Closing Remarks

As we close the final chapter of this journey together, we hope that the lessons gleaned, the stories recounted and the wisdom imparted will serve as a continuous source of inspiration, provocation and guidance.

By implementing the principles and practices outlined in *Essential Skills for Physiotherapists*, you will not only enrich your own existence but also profoundly affect the lives of your patients, your friends and your family – as well as the bigger international physiotherapy community.

From picking up this book and reading it, you are already striving to improve.

To become better. And never let this desire stop.

Never stop learning.

Keep asking questions.

Stay curious, that little bit longer, as Michael Bungay Stanier (2020) says.

Be 'The Learning Physiotherapist'.

References

Brown, B. (2019). *Dare to lead: Brave work, tough conversations, whole hearts*. New York: Random House Large Print.

Burkeman, O. (2022). *Four thousand weeks: Embrace your limits. Change your life. Make your four thousand weeks count*. Vintage.

Caroselli, M. (2000). *Leadership skills for managers*. McGraw-Hill Education.

Greene, R. (2012). *Mastery*. Profile Books.

Hamburger, P. (1952, December 13). *Men of faith. The New Yorker Magazine Inc.*, pp. 167–169 (Online New Yorker archive of digital scans).

Heath, C., & Heath, D. (2007). *Made to stick: Why some ideas survive and others die*. Random House.

Kerr, J. (2013). *Legacy: What the All Blacks can teach us about the business of life*. Constable.

Kotler, S. (2014). *The rise of Superman: Decoding the science of ultimate human performance*. Houghton Mifflin Harcourt.

Pressfield, S. (2002). *The war of art: Break through the blocks and win your inner creative battles*. Black Irish Entertainment LLC.

Robbins, M. (11 June 2011). How to stop screwing yourself over. TEDxSF. [Video]. YouTube. Available at https://www.youtube.com/watch?v=Lp7E973zozc&t=32s&ab_channel=TEDxTalks.

Bungay Stanier, M. B. (2020). *Advice trap: Be humble, stay curious and change the way you lead forever*. Page Two Books, Inc.

Walsh, B. (2010). *The score takes care of itself: My philosophy of leadership*. Penguin Publishing Group.

Note: Page numbers followed by *f* indicate figures and *t* indicate tables.